Fourth Edition

Registered Health Information Administrator (RHIA) Exam Preparation

Patricia Shaw,
MEd, RHIA, FAHIMA

and

Darcy Carter,
MHA, RHIA

Editors

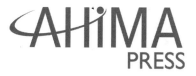

D1474394

ISBN: 978-1-58426-386-9

AHIMA Product No. AB106012

AHIMA Staff:
Jessica Block, MA, Assistant Editor
Angie Comfort, RHIT, CCS, Technical Review
Katie Greenock, MS, Editorial and Production Coordinator
Jason O. Malley, Director, Creative Content Development
Lou Ann Wiedemann, MS, RHIA, FAHIMA, CPEHR, Technical Review
Pamela Woolf, Managing Editor

For more information, including updates, about AHIMA Press publications, visit http://www.ahima.org/publications/updates.aspx.

American Health Information Management Association
233 North Michigan Avenue, 21st Floor
Chicago, Illinois 60601-5809
ahima.org

Contents

On the Website

Practice Questions with Answers
Practice Exam 1 with Answers
Practice Exam 2 with Answers
Practice Exam 3 with Answers (*Bonus Exam*)
Health Information Management Glossary e-flashcards (4,500+ terms)
Hospital Statistical Formulas Used for the RHIA Exam

About the Editors

Patricia Shaw, MEd, RHIA, FAHIMA, earned her master's degree in education in 1997 and is currently working on a Doctorate degree in Education. Ms. Shaw has been on the faculty of Weber State University since 1991, where she teaches in the health information management and health services administration programs. She has primary teaching responsibility for the quality and performance improvement, coding, reimbursement, and data management curriculum in those programs. Ms. Shaw maintains contact with practice settings as a consultant specializing in the areas of reimbursement and coding issues. Prior to accepting a position at Weber State University, Ms. Shaw managed hospital health information services departments and was a nosologist for 3M Health Information Systems.

Darcy Carter, MHA, RHIA, earned her master's degree in healthcare administration and is currently pursuing a doctorate degree in health sciences. She is on the faculty in the health information management and technology programs at Weber State University, where she teaches courses in coding, reimbursement, and database management for the programs. Ms. Carter also continues to work as a coder/abstractor at McKay-Dee Hospital Center.

About the RHIA Exam

Job opportunities for RHIAs exist in multiple settings throughout the healthcare industry. These include the continuum of care delivery organizations, including hospitals, multispecialty clinics and physician practices, long-term care, mental health, and other ambulatory care settings. The profession has seen significant expansion in nonpatient care settings, with careers in managed care and insurance companies, software vendors, consulting services, government agencies, education, and pharmaceutical companies.

Working as a critical link between care providers, payers, and patients, an RHIA:

- Is an expert in managing patient health information and medical records, administering computer information systems, collecting and analyzing patient data, and using classification systems and medical terminologies
- Possesses comprehensive knowledge of medical, administrative, ethical, and legal requirements and standards related to healthcare delivery and the privacy of protected patient information
- Manages people and operational units, participates in administrative committees, and prepares budgets
- Interacts with all levels of an organization—clinical, financial, administrative, and information systems—that employ patient data in decision-making and everyday operations

The National Commission for Certifying Agencies (NCCA) has granted accreditation to AHIMA's Registered Health Information Administrator (RHIA) certification program. This accomplishment establishes AHIMA as the industry leader in accredited health information and informatics management (HIIM) certification programs, and advances AHIMA's organizational mission of positioning AHIMA members and certificants as recognized leaders in advancing professional practice and standards in HIIM.

The Commission on Certification for Health Informatics and Information Management (CCHIIM) manages and sets the strategic direction for the certifications. Pearson Vue is the exclusive provider of AHIMA certification exams. To see sample questions and images of the new exam format, visit ahima.org/certification. For more detailed information, including eligibility requirements, visit ahima.org/certification.

Exam Competency Statements

A certification exam is based on an explicit set of competencies. These competencies have been determined through a job analysis study conducted of practitioners. The competencies are subdivided into domains and tasks, as listed here. Each domain is allocated a predefined number of questions at specific cognitive levels to make up the exam. The RHIA exam tests only content pertaining to the following competencies.

Domain I: Health Data Management (20% of exam)

1. Manage health data elements and/or data sets.
2. Develop and maintain organizational policies, procedures, and guidelines for management of health information.
3. Ensure accuracy and integrity of health data and health record documentation.
4. Manage and/or validate coding accuracy and compliance.

5. Manage the use of clinical data required in reimbursement systems and prospective payment systems (PPS) in healthcare delivery.
6. Code diagnosis and procedures according to established guidelines.
7. Present data for organizational use (for example, summarize, synthesize, and condense information).

Domain II: Health Statistics and Research Support (11% of exam)

1. Identify and/or respond to the information needs of internal and external healthcare customers.
2. Filter and/or interpret information for the end customer.
3. Analyze and present information for organizational management (for example, quality, utilization, risk).
4. Use data mining techniques to query and report from databases.

Domain III: Information Technology and Systems (20% of exam)

1. Implement and manage use of technology applications.
2. Develop data dictionary and data models for database design.
3. Manage and maintain databases (for example, data migration and updates).
4. Apply data and functional standards to achieve interoperability of healthcare information systems.
5. Apply data/record storage principles and techniques associated with the medium (for example, paper-based, hybrid, electronic).
6. Evaluate and recommend clinical, administrative, and specialty service applications (for example, financial systems, electronic record, clinical coding).
7. Manage master person index (for example, patient record integration, customer/client relationship management).

Domain IV: Organization and Management (30% of exam)

1. Develop and support strategic and operational plans for facility-wide health information management.
2. Monitor industry trends and organizational needs to anticipate changes.
3. Perform human resource management activities (for example, recruiting staff, creating job descriptions, resolve personnel issues).
4. Conduct training and educational activities (for example, HIM systems, coding, medical and institutional terminology; documentation and regulatory requirements).
5. Establish and monitor productivity standards for the HIM function.
6. Optimize reimbursement through management of the revenue cycle (for example, Chargemaster maintenance).
7. Develop, motivate, and support work teams and/or individuals (for example, coaching, mentoring).
8. Prepare and manage budgets.
9. Analyze and report on budget variances.
10. Determine resource needs by performing analyses (for example, cost-benefit, business planning).

11. Evaluate and manage contracts (for example, vendor, contract personnel, maintenance).
12. Organize and facilitate meetings.
13. Advocate for department, organization, and/or profession.
14. Manage projects.
15. Prepare for accreditation and licensing processes (for example, the Joint Commission, Medicare, state regulators).

Domain V: Privacy, Security, and Confidentiality (13% of exam)

1. Design and implement security measures to safeguard protected health information (PHI).
2. Manage access, disclosure, and use of PHI to ensure confidentiality.
3. Investigate and resolve healthcare privacy and security issues and problems.
4. Develop and maintain healthcare privacy and security training programs.

Domain VI: Legal and Regulatory Standards (6% of exam)

1. Administer organizational compliance with healthcare information laws, regulations, and standards (for example, audit, report and/or inform; legal health record).
2. Prepare for accreditation and licensing processes (for example, the Joint Commission, Medicare, state regulators).

RHIA Exam Specifications

The RHIA is made up of 180 four-option, multiple choice questions. The computer will monitor the time you spend on the exam. A clock in the upper-right corner of the screen will indicate the time remaining to complete the exam. The exam will terminate at the allotted time limit—4 hours.

During the exam, formulas for commonly used healthcare rates and percentages will be provided only for items for which they are needed. These formulas are also listed on page 246 in the back of this book. A calculator will also be available during the exam.

ICD-9-CM, CPT, and HCPCS coding concepts will be tested on the RHIA exam. However, coding books will not be needed to take the exam. All necessary information needed to answer a coding question will be included as part of the question. This will include the code, narrative, and other information that may need to be reproduced from the codebooks. Commonly used formulas will also be provided as necessary for specific exam questions. For more RHIA exam information, visit ahima.org/certification.

How to Use This Book

The RHIA practice questions and exams in this book and on the accompanying website test knowledge of content pertaining to the RHIA competencies published by AHIMA.

The multiple choice practice questions and exams in this book and its companion website are presented in a similar format to those that might be found on the RHIA exam. The book contains 460 multiple choice practice questions and two practice exams (with 180 questions each). Because each question is organized by and identified with one of the six RHIA domains, you will be able to determine whether you need knowledge or skill building in particular areas of the exam domains. Each answer includes a rationale and reference. Pursuing the sources of these references will help you build your knowledge and skills in specific domains.

To effectively use this book, work through all of the practice questions first. This will help you identify areas in which you may need further preparation. For the questions that you answer incorrectly, read the associated references to help refresh your knowledge. After going through the practice questions, take one of the practice exams. Again, for the questions that you answer incorrectly, refresh your knowledge by reading the associated references. Continue in the same manner with the second exam and third practice exam. (Practice Exam 3 is a bonus web-based exam.)

Retake the practice questions and exams as many times as you like. To help build your knowledge and skills, you should review the references provided for all questions that you answered incorrectly.

The accompanying website for *RHIA Exam Preparation,* Fourth Edition, contains 1,000 questions—the same 460 practice questions and two practice exams printed in the book and a bonus practice exam. Each of the self-scoring exams can be run in practice mode—which allows you to work at your own pace—or exam mode—which simulates the four-hour timed exam experience. The practice questions and simulated exams on the web can be set to be presented in random order, or you may choose to go through the questions in sequential order by domain. You may also choose to practice or test your skills on specific domains. For example, if you would like to build your skills in domain III, you may choose only domain III questions for a given practice session.

The website also includes a glossary of electronic flashcards for 4,500+ health information management-related terms and definitions as well as a listing of commonly used formulas that are available to test takers during the RHIA exam.

PRACTICE QUESTIONS

Domain I   *Health Data Management*

1. What term is used in reference to objective descriptions of processes, procedures, people, and other observable objects and activities?

   a. Information

   b. Data

   c. Knowledge

   d. Notices

2. Which of the following processes is an ancillary function of the health record?

   a. Medical error prevention

   b. Data and information storage

   c. Patient assessment and care planning

   d. Biomedical research

3. What term is used in reference to electronically accessed information that provides physicians with pertinent health information beyond the health record itself?

   a. Core measures

   b. Advanced decision support

   c. Clinical practice guidelines

   d. Enhanced discharge planning

4. To which of the following authorities do hospitals report vital statistics?

   a. World Health Organization

   b. National Vital Statistics System

   c. Centers for Disease Control

   d. The designated state authority

5. An attempt to contain hospital inpatient costs and improve quality by restructuring services is called:

   a. Continuous quality improvement

   b. Patient-focused care

   c. Managed care

   d. Acute care

6. What organization was established in 1847 to represent the interests of physicians across the United States?

   a. American Association of Medical Colleges

   b. American College of Surgeons

   c. Committee on Medical Education

   d. American Medical Association

7. Today, to practice medicine, medical school students must pass a test before they can obtain a:

   a. Degree

   b. Residency

   c. Specialty

   d. License

8. For healthcare organizations, this modern process began with the adoption of the Minimum Standards:

   a. Accreditation

   b. Licensing

   c. Reform

   d. Educational

9. Which process requires the verification of the educational qualifications, licensure status, and other experience of healthcare professionals who have applied for the privilege of practicing within a healthcare facility?

   a. Deemed status

   b. Judicial decision

   c. Subpoena

   d. Credentialing

10. Which of the following is a mechanism that records and examines activity in information systems?

    a. eSignature laws

    b. Audit controls

    c. Minimum necessary rules

    d. Access controls

11. Which of the following is the goal of quantitative analysis performed by HIM professionals?

    a. Ensuring the record is legible

    b. Identifying deficiencies early so they can be completed

    c. Verifying that health professionals are providing appropriate care

    d. Checking to ensure bills are correct

12. What are LOINC codes used for?

    a. Identifying test results

    b. Reporting test results

    c. Identifying tests unique to a specific company

    d. Reporting a code for reimbursement

13. While the focus of inpatient data collection is on the principal diagnosis, the focus of outpatient data collection is on the:

    a. Reason for admission

    b. Reason for encounter

    c. Discharge diagnosis

    d. Activities of daily living

14. The inpatient data set incorporated into federal law and required for Medicare reporting is the:

    a. Ambulatory Care Data Set

    b. Uniform Hospital Discharge Data Set

    c. Minimum Data Set for Long-term Care

    d. Health Plan Employer Data and Information Set

15. In order to effectively transmit healthcare data between a provider and payer, both parties must adhere to which electronic data interchange standards?

    a. X12N

    b. LOINC

    c. IEEE 1073

    d. DICOM

16. This document is a snapshot of a patient's status and includes everything from social issues to disease processes as well as critical paths and clinical pathways that focus on a specific disease process or pathway in an LTCH.

    a. Face sheet

    b. Care plan

    c. Diagnosis plan

    d. Flow sheet

17. Which of the following is a component of the Resident Assessment Instrument?

    a. The resident's health record

    b. A standard Minimum Data Set (MDS)

    c. Preadmission Screening Assessment

    d. Annual Resident Review

18. Which of the following personnel should be authorized, per hospital policy, to take a physician's verbal order for the administration of medication?

    a. Unit secretary working on the unit where the patient is located

    b. Nurse working on the unit where the patient is located

    c. Health information director

    d. Admissions registrars

19. Who is responsible for ensuring the quality of health record documentation?

    a. Board of directors

    b. Administrator

    c. Provider

    d. Health information management professional

20. Of the following, what is the most likely to happen to the health records of a physician's patient when a physician leaves an office practice?

    a. It will be sent to the state department of health.

    b. It will be sent to outside storage.

    c. It will be destroyed.

    d. It will be retained by the practice.

21. Which health record format is arranged in chronological order with documentation from various sources intermingled?

    a. Electronic

    b. Source-oriented

    c. Problem-oriented

    d. Integrated

22. Staff disagreements within the health record should be:

    a. Avoided

    b. Detailed and thorough

    c. Included in incident reports

    d. Documented according to state regulations

23. Mrs. Bolton is an angry patient who resents her physicians "bossing her around." She refuses to take a portion of the medications the nurses bring to her pursuant to physician orders and is verbally abusive to the patient care assistants. Of the following options, the most appropriate way to document Mrs. Bolton's behavior in the patient health record is:

    a. Mean

    b. Noncompliant and hostile toward staff

    c. Belligerent and out of line

    d. A pain in the neck

24. The _____ is/are used to complete comprehensive assessments and collect information for the Minimum Data Set for Long-term Care (MDS).

    a. Resident Assessment Protocols

    b. Resident Assessment Instrument

    c. Utilization guidelines

    d. Minimum Data Set

25. One technology used for computer-assisted coding is:

    a. Logic-based encoding

    b. Natural language processing

    c. Artificial intelligence

    d. Coder intervention

26. A barrier to effective computer-assisted coding is the:

    a. Resistance of physicians

    b. Resistance of HIM professionals

    c. Poor quality of documentation

    d. Reduction of consistency without human coders

27. According to the UHDDS definition, ethnicity should be recorded on a patient record as:

    a. Race of mother

    b. Race of father

    c. Spanish origin/Hispanic, non-Spanish origin/non-Hispanic, unknown

    d. Free-text descriptor as reported by patient

28. A coding supervisor checks coding quality each month by having two or more coders code the same set of records and then comparing the results. This process addresses the data quality element of:

    a. Validity

    b. Granularity

    c. Timeliness

    d. Reliability

29. A core data set developed by ASTM to communicate a patient's past and current health information as the patient's transitions from one care setting to another is:

    a. Continuity of Care Record

    b. Minimum Data Set

    c. Ambulatory Care Data Set

    d. Uniform Hospital Discharge Data Set

30. A consumer interested in comparing the performance of health plans should review data from:

    a. HEDIS

    b. OASIS

    c. ORYX

    d. UHDDS

31. Changes and updates to ICD-9-CM are managed by the ICD-9-CM Coordination and Maintenance Committee, a federal committee co-chaired by representatives from the NCHS and:

    a. AMA

    b. OIG

    c. CMS

    d. WHO

32. A computer software program that supports a coder in assigning correct codes is called a(n):

    a. Encoder

    b. Grouper

    c. Automated coder

    d. Decision support system

33. Diagnosis described as "possible," "probable," "likely," or "rule out" is reported as if present for which type of patient records?

    a. Outpatient

    b. Emergency room

    c. Physician office

    d. Inpatient

34. Patient has HIV with disseminated candidiasis; what is the correct code assignment?

042	Human immunodeficiency virus [HIV] disease
112.0	Candidiasis of mouth
112.5	Candidiasis, disseminated
112.89	Candidiasis, of other specified sites, other

    a. 042, 112.0

    b. 112.5, 042

    c. 042, 112.5

    d. 042, 112.89, 112.5

35. A 65-year-old woman was admitted to the hospital. She was diagnosed with septicemia secondary to staphylococcus aureus and abdominal pain secondary to diverticulitis of the colon. What is the correct code assignment?

038.11	Methicillin susceptible *Staphylococcus Aureus* septicemia
038.8	Other specified septicemia
038.9	Unspecified septicemia
041.11	Methicillin susceptible staphylococcus aureus
562.11	Diverticulitis of colon (without mention of hemorrhage)
789.00	Abdominal pain, unspecified site

    a. 038.8, 562.11, 789.00

    b. 038.11, 562.11

    c. 038.8, 562.11, 041.11

    d. 038.9, 562.11

36. Patient was admitted to the hospital and diagnosed with diabetic gangrene. What is the correct code assignment?

250.00	Diabetes mellitus without mention of complication, type II or unspecified type, not stated as uncontrolled	
250.70	Diabetes with peripheral circulatory disorders, type II or unspecified type, not stated as uncontrolled	
250.71	Diabetes with peripheral circulatory disorders, type I [juvenile type], not stated as uncontrolled	
785.4	Gangrene	

    a. 250.71, 785.4

    b. 785.4, 250.70

    c. 250.70, 250.00, 785.4

    d. 250.70, 785.4

37. Patient had carcinoma of the anterior bladder wall fulgurated three years ago. The patient returns yearly for a cystoscopy to recheck for bladder tumor. The patient is currently admitted for a routine check. A small recurring malignancy is found and fulgurated during the cystoscopy procedure. What is the correct code assignment?

188.3	Malignant neoplasm of bladder, anterior wall of urinary bladder
198.1	Secondary malignant neoplasm of other specified sites, other urinary organs
V10.51	Personal history of malignant neoplasm, bladder
57.32	Diagnostic procedure on bladder, other cystoscopy
57.49	Other transurethral excision or destruction of lesion or tissue of bladder

    a. 188.3, V10.51, 57.49, 57.32

    b. 198.1, 57.49

    c. 188.3, 57.49

    d. 198.1, 188.3, 57.49

38. A patient with a diagnosis of ventral hernia is admitted to undergo a laparotomy with ventral hernia repair. The patient undergoes a laparotomy and develops bradycardia. The operative site is closed without the repair of the hernia. What is the correct code assignment?

427.89	Other specified cardiac dysrhythmias, other
553.20	Ventral hernia, unspecified
997.1	Complications affecting specified body systems, not elsewhere classified, cardiac complications
V64.1	Surgical or other procedure not carried out because of contraindication
54.11	Exploratory laparotomy
54.19	Other laparotomy

    a. 553.20, 427.89, V64.1, 54.19

    b. 553.20, 997.1, 427.89, 54.19

    c. 553.20, 54.11

    d. 553.20, 54.11, V64.1

39. These codes are used to assign a diagnosis to a patient who is seeking health services but is not necessarily sick.

    a. E codes

    b. V codes

    c. M codes

    d. C codes

40. Patient was admitted through the emergency department following a fall from a ladder while painting his house. He had contusions of the scalp and face and an open fracture of the intracapsular section of the left femur. The fracture site was debrided and the fracture was reduced by open procedure, with an external fixation device applied. What is the correct code assignment?

820.00	Fracture of neck of femur, transcervical fracture, closed, intracapsular section, unspecified
820.10	Fracture of neck of femur, transcervical fracture, open, intracapsular section, unspecified
920	Contusion of face, scalp, and neck except eye(s)
E881.0	Fall from ladder
E849.0	Place of occurrence, home
E016.9	Other activity involving property and land maintenance, building and construction
E000.8	External cause status, specified NEC
78.15	Application of external fixator device, femur
79.25	Open reduction of fracture without internal fixation, femur
79.35	Open reduction of fracture with internal fixation, femur
79.65	Debridement of open fracture site, femur

    a. 820.00, E881.0, E849.0, E000.8, 79.25, 78.15

    b. 820.10, 920, E881.0, E849.0, E016.9, E000.8, 79.25, 78.15, 79.65

    c. 820.00, E881.0, 79.35, 79.65

    d. 820.10, E881.0, E849.0, E016.9, E000.8, 79.25, 78.15, 79.65

41. Assign the correct CPT code for the following procedure: Revision of the pacemaker skin pocket.

    a. 33223, Revision of skin pocket for cardioverter-defibrillator

    b. 33210, Insertion or replacement of temporary transvenous single chamber cardiac electrode or pacemaker catheter (separate procedure)

    c. 33212, Insertion of pacemaker pulse generator only; with existing single lead

    d. 33222, Revision or relocation of skin pocket for pacemaker

42. Assign the correct CPT code for the following: A 63-year-old female had a temporal artery biopsy completed in the outpatient surgical center.

    a. 32405, Biopsy, lung or mediastinum, percutaneous needle

    b. 37609, Ligation or biopsy, temporal artery

    c. 20206, Biopsy, muscle, percutaneous needle

    d. 31629, Bronchoscopy, rigid or flexible, with or without fluoroscopic guidance when performed; with transbronchial needle aspiration biopsy(s), trachea, mainstem and/or lobar bronchus(i)

43. Assign the correct CPT code for the following: A 58-year-old male was seen in the outpatient surgical center for insertion of a self-contained inflatable penile prosthesis for impotence.

    a. 54401, Insertion of penile prosthesis; inflatable (self-contained)

    b. 54405, Insertion of multi-component, inflatable penile prosthesis, including placement of pump, cylinders, and reservoir

    c. 54440, Plastic operation of penis for injury

    d. 54400, Insertion of penile prosthesis, non-inflatable (semi-rigid)

44. A patient returns during a 90-day postoperative period from a ventral hernia repair; the patient is now complaining of eye pain. What modifier would you use with the Evaluation and Management code?

    a. −79, Unrelated procedure or service by the same physician during the postoperative period

    b. −25, Significant, separately identifiable evaluation and management service by the same physician on the same day of the procedure or other service

    c. −59, Distinct procedural service

    d. −24, Unrelated evaluation and management service by the same physician during a postoperative period

45. Medicaid coverage is not identical in New Jersey, California, or Idaho. Which of the following reasons is correct?

    a. Federal funds allocated to each state are based on the size of the state.

    b. The program must cover infants born to Medicaid-eligible pregnant women.

    c. States that offer an SCHIP program do not have a Medicaid program.

    d. Medicaid allows states to maintain a unique program adapted to state residents' needs and average incomes.

46. Which TRICARE program offers services to active duty family members (ADFMs) with no enrollment, deductible, or copayment fees for covered services?

    a. TRICARE Prime

    b. TRICARE Standard

    c. TRICARE for Life

    d. TRICARE Plus

47. Under RBRVS which elements are used to calculate a Medicare payment?

    a. Work value and extent of the physical exam

    b. Malpractice expenses and detail of the patient history

    c. Work value and practice expenses

    d. Practice expenses and review of systems

48. What is the average of the sum of the relative weights of all patients treated during a specified time period?

    a. Case-mix index

    b. Outlier pool

    c. Share

    d. Mean qualifier

49. Medicare's payment system for home health services consolidates all types of services, such as speech, physical, and occupational therapy, into a single lump-sum payment. What type of healthcare payment method does this lump-sum payment represent?

    a. Global payment

    b. Capitated rate

    c. Customary, prevailing, and reasonable

    d. Resource-based relative value scale

50. In terms of grouping and reimbursement, how are the MS-LTC-DRGs and acute-care MS-DRGs similar?

    a. Relative weights

    b. Based on principal diagnosis

    c. Categorization of low-volume groups into quintiles

    d. Classification of short-stay outliers

51. In the LTCH PPS, what is the standard federal rate?

    a. Constant that converts the MS-LTC-DRG weight into a payment

    b. Relative weight based on the market basket of goods

    c. Geographic wage index

    d. Adjustment mandated by the Benefits Improvement and Protection Act (BIPA) of 2000

52. To meet the definition of an inpatient rehabilitation facility (IRF), facilities must have an inpatient population with at least a specified percentage of patients with certain conditions. Which of the following conditions is counted in the definition?

    a. Brain injury

    b. Chronic myelogenous leukemia

    c. Acute myocardial infarction

    d. Cancer

53. It is the year 201X. The federal government is determined to lower the overall payments to physicians. To incur the least administrative work, which of the following elements of the physician payment system would the government reduce?

    a. Conversion factor

    b. RVU

    c. GPCI

    d. Weighted discount

54. In the HHPPS system, which home healthcare services are consolidated into a single payment to home health agencies?

    a. Home health aide visits, routine and nonroutine medical supplies, durable medical equipment

    b. Routine and nonroutine medical supplies, durable medical equipment, medical social services

    c. Nursing and therapy services, routine and nonroutine medical supplies, home health aide visits

    d. Nursing and therapy services, durable medical equipment, medical social services

55. Which of the following items are packaged under the Medicare hospital outpatient prospective payment system (HOPPS)?

    a. Recovery room and medical visits

    b. Medical visits and supplies (other than pass-through)

    c. Anesthesia and ambulance services

    d. Supplies (other than pass-through) and recovery room

56. Which of the following statements is true about APCs?

    a. APCs are based solely on the patient's principal diagnosis.

    b. ICD-9-CM procedure codes are used to group patients.

    c. Severity of illness is taken into consideration when grouping APCs.

    d. APCs are based on the CPT or HCPCS code(s) reported.

57. In the APC system, an outlier payment is paid when which of the following occurs?

    a. The cost of the service is greater than the APC payment by a fixed ratio and exceeds the APC payment plus a threshold amount.

    b. The LOS is greater than expected.

    c. The charges for the services provided are greater than the expected payment.

    d. The total cost of all the services is greater than the sum of APC payments by a fixed ratio and exceeds the sum of APC payments plus a threshold amount.

58. This PPS has been adopted for use by many third-party payers (for example, Medicaid) for reimbursement of outpatient visits. It is not the methodology used by Medicare.

    a. ASCs (ambulatory surgical centers)

    b. APGs (ambulatory patient groups)

    c. DRGs (diagnosis-related groups)

    d. APCs (ambulatory payment classifications)

59. The Omnibus Budget Reconciliation Act of 1980 amended the SSA to specify which procedures would be covered under the prospective payment system for ambulatory surgical centers. This PPS is officially named the ASC _____.

    a. List of Covered Procedures

    b. List of Covered Surgeries

    c. Fee Schedule

    d. PPS

60. Which of the following conditions are included on the hospital-acquired conditions provision list?

    a. Pressure ulcers, staphylococcus infections, gunshot wounds

    b. Staphylococcus infections, air embolism, physical and substance abuse

    c. Catheter associated urinary tract infections, gunshot wounds

    d. Pressure ulcers, catheter associated urinary tract infections, falls and fractures

61. Long-term acute care is paid under which of the following Medicare systems?

    a. SNF Resource Utilization Groups (RUGS)

    b. Medicare Inpatient Rehabilitation Facilities (IRF)

    c. Medicare prospective payment system (PPS)

    d. Medicare Severity Diagnostic-Related Groups (MS-DRGs)

62. If an HIM employee acts in deliberate ignorance or in disregard to official coding guidelines, it may constitute:

    a. Abuse

    b. Fraud

    c. Malpractice

    d. Kickbacks

63. If an HIM department receives gifts from vendors in exchange for purchasing a specific encoder software, this is:

    a. Abuse

    b. Negligence

    c. Malpractice

    d. A kickback

64. Exceptions to the Federal Anti-Kickback Statute that allow legitimate business arrangements and are not subject to prosecution are:

    a. *Qui tam* practices

    b. Safe practices

    c. Safe harbors

    d. Exclusions

65. The federal physician self-referral statute is also known as the:

    a. Sherman Anti-Trust Act

    b. Deficit Reduction Act

    c. False Claims Act

    d. Stark Law

66. According to the OIG, insufficient or missing documentation and which one of the following are responsible for 70 percent of bad claims submitted to Medicare?

    a. Local coverage decisions

    b. Unbundling of procedures

    c. Failure to document medical necessity

    d. Overcoding

67. The combination of certain items (such as anesthesia, supplies, and drugs) for the purpose of reimbursement is called:

    a. Packaging

    b. Discounting

    c. Rate setting

    d. Case mix

68. Which of the following is a generic term for a healthcare reimbursement system that manages cost, quality, and access to services?

    a. Quality improvement

    b. Subacute care

    c. Managed care

    d. Patient-focused care

69. What is the term for an index based on relative differences in the cost of a market basket of goods across areas?

    a. Bundle

    b. CPI

    c. GPCI

    d. Cost-to-charge

70. Using the information provided, if the physician is a non-PAR who accepts assignment, how much can he or she expect to be reimbursed by Medicare?

> Physician's normal charge = $340
> Medicare Fee Schedule = $300
> Patient has met his deductible.

    a. $228

    b. $240

    c. $285

    d. $300

Use the following figure for questions 71 through 75:

```
┌─────────────────────────────────────────┐
│          ABC Premiere Health Plan         │
├───────────────────────────────────────────┤
│  MEMBER                  POLICY NUMBER     │
│  JANE B. WHITE           HS 123456 7890    │
│                                            │
│  GROUP                                     │
│  STATE                                     │
│                                            │
│  TYPE                    EFFEC 01012005    │
│  EMPLOYEE-ONLY                             │
│                                            │
│  SEND ALL BILLS TO:                        │
│  ABC Premiere Health Plan                  │
│  1500 Primrose Path                        │
│  Flowerville, XX 12345                     │
└────────────────────────────────────────────┘
```

71. From the figure, determine the subscriber.

    a. STATE

    b. ABC Premiere Health Plan

    c. JANE B. WHITE

    d. Cannot be determined

72. From the figure, determine whether the plan covers Gill F. White, Jane's spouse.

    a. No; the card states "Employee-Only."

    b. Yes; the policy number includes "S."

    c. Yes; the group is "State."

    d. Cannot be determined.

73. What third-party payer does the figure represent?

    a. Medicaid

    b. Medicare

    c. Blue Cross and Blue Shield

    d. Commercial healthcare insurance

74. According to the figure, what type of coverage does the third-party payer provide Jane B. White?

    a. Family

    b. Dependent

    c. Individual

    d. Premiere

75. From the figure, determine who is the entity that has purchased the insurance policy.

    a. 1234567890

    b. STATE

    c. ABC Premiere Health Plan

    d. Jane B. White

76. What is ISO 9000?

    a. A set of financial standards of accounting to which all organizations must conform

    b. A European company that has set the standard for excellence in strategic planning

    c. The newest information management system allowing decision makers to monitor all organizational databases

    d. A set of international standards for quality management

77. Which of the following are considered vital records?

    a. Birth, marriage, and late fetal death

    b. Birth, registry, and adoption

    c. Marriage, divorce, and registry

    d. Late fetal death, passport, and birth

78. Mary Smith, RHIA, has been charged with the responsibility of designing a data collection form to be used on admission of a patient to the acute-care hospital in which she works. What is the first resource she should use?

    a. UHDDS

    b. UACDS

    c. MDS

    d. ORYX

79. What is the traditional format for a hospital patient care record?

    a. Integrated

    b. Practice-oriented

    c. Chronological

    d. Source-oriented

80. Which of the following govern(s) the operation of a hospital medical staff?

    a. Medical staff classification

    b. Medical staff bylaws

    c. Medical staff credentialing

    d. Medical staff committees

81. Medical staff bylaws are legally binding and any changes must be approved by a vote of which of the following?

    a. Hospital staff

    b. Administrative staff

    c. Hospital attorney

    d. Medical staff

82. What classification of medical staff membership denies admitting privileges but recognizes the contributions and reputations of its members?

    a. Active

    b. Honorary

    c. Courtesy

    d. Affiliate

83. Which of the following is required in order to prescribe medications?

    a. Active medical staff membership

    b. A drug enforcement agency number

    c. A position on a medical staff executive committee

    d. A credential from a nationally recognized association

84. In data quality management, the processes and systems used to archive data and data journals are called:

    a. Collection

    b. Warehousing

    c. Application

    d. Analysis

85. Which of the following are considered dimensions of data quality?

    a. Relevancy, granularity, timeliness, currency, accuracy, precision, and consistency

    b. Relevancy, granularity, timeliness, currency, atomic, precision, and consistency

    c. Relevancy, granularity, timeliness, concurrent, atomic, precision, and consistency

    d. Relevancy, granularity, equality, currency, precision, accuracy, and consistency

86. Define a fetal death.

    a. Death of a fetus of 500 g or more

    b. Death of a fetus of 22 or more weeks of gestation

    c. Death of a fetus declared a fetal death by the physician

    d. Death of a fetus of a weight and week gestation determined by state law

87. Which of the following must be reported to the medical examiner?

    a. Burns

    b. Accidental deaths

    c. Causes of injury

    d. Morbidity

88. Which of the following generally describes a coroner and a medical examiner, both of whom examine suspicious deaths?

    a. Medical examiner is usually a nonphysician elected official; coroner is appointed.

    b. Medical examiner is a pathologist; coroner is not a physician.

    c. Medical examiner is appointed by the court; coroner is a physician.

    d. Medical examiner is usually a physician; coroner is appointed or elected and may or may not be a physician.

89. In figuring a drug dosage, it is unacceptable to round up to the nearest gram if the drug is to be dosed in milligrams. Which dimension of data quality is being applied in this situation?

    a. Accuracy

    b. Granularity

    c. Precision

    d. Currency

90. A patient's name is typically stored in a database as three data elements—last name, first name, and middle name—and not as a single data element. Which dimension of data quality is being applied when this occurs?

    a. Accuracy

    b. Granularity

    c. Precision

    d. Currency

Domain II *Health Statistics and Research Support*

91. The Tax Relief and Health Care Act of 2006 (MIEA-TRHCA) expanded CMS quality initiatives to which two settings?

    a. Skilled nursing facilities and ambulatory surgical centers

    b. Hospital outpatient departments and ambulatory surgical centers

    c. Hospital outpatient departments and physician group practices

    d. Skilled nursing facilities and physician group practices

92. The researcher mined the Medicare Provider Analysis Review (MEDPAR) file. The analysis revealed trends in lengths of stay for rural hospitals. What type of investigation was the researcher conducting?

    a. Content analysis

    b. Effect size review

    c. Psychometric assay

    d. Secondary analysis

93. Which of the following terms is defined as the proportion of people in a population who have a particular disease at a specific point in time or over a specified period of time?

    a. Prevalence

    b. Incidence

    c. Frequency

    d. Distribution

94. The foundations of care giving, which include buildings, equipment, professional staff, and appropriate policies are included in what area of performance measurement?

    a. Outcomes

    b. Processes

    c. Systems

    d. Benchmarks

95. The interrelated activities in healthcare organizations that promote effective and safe patient outcomes across services and disciplines within an integrated environment are included in what area of performance measurement?

    a. Outcomes

    b. Processes

    c. Systems

    d. Benchmarks

96. The final results of care, treatment, and services in terms of the patient's expectations, needs, and quality of life, which may be positive and appropriate or negative and diminishing, are included in what area of performance measurement?

    a. Outcomes

    b. Processes

    c. Systems

    d. Benchmarks

97. This type of performance measure focuses on a process that leads to a certain outcome, meaning that a scientific basis exists for believing that the process, when executed well, will increase the probability of achieving a desired outcome.

    a. Outcome measure

    b. Data measure

    c. Process measure

    d. System measure

98. This type of performance measure indicates the result of the performance or nonperformance of a function or process.

    a. Outcome measure

    b. Data measure

    c. Process measure

    d. System measure

99. The percent of antibiotics administered immediately prior to open reduction and internal fixation (ORIF) surgeries or the percent of deliveries accomplished by cesarean section are examples of what type of performance measure?

    a. Outcome measure

    b. Data measure

    c. Process measure

    d. System measure

100. This data collection tool is used when one needs to gather data on sample observations in order to detect patterns.

    a. Check sheet

    b. Ordinal data tool

    c. Balance sheet

    d. Nominal data tool

101. This type of data is also called categorical data and includes values assigned to name-specific categories.

    a. Nominal data

    b. Ordinal data

    c. Discrete data

    d. Continuous data

102. This type of data is also called ranked data and expresses the comparative evaluation of various characteristics or entities, and relative assignment of each, to a class according to a set of criteria.

    a. Nominal data

    b. Ordinal data

    c. Discrete data

    d. Continuous data

103. This type of data is numerical values that represent whole numbers.

    a. Nominal data

    b. Ordinal data

    c. Discrete data

    d. Continuous data

104. This type of data assumes an infinite number of possible values in measurements that have decimal values as possibilities.

    a. Nominal data

    b. Ordinal data

    c. Discrete data

    d. Continuous data

105. A research instrument that is used to gather data and information from respondents in a uniform manner through the administration of a predefined and structured set of questions and possible responses is called a(n):

    a. Survey

    b. Interview

    c. Process measure

    d. Affinity diagram

106. In this type of interview the sequence of questions is not planned in advance and is conducted in a friendly, conversational manner.

    a. Structured interview

    b. Unstructured interview

    c. Planned interview

    d. Unplanned interview

107. In this type of interview, a predetermined list of questions is used.

    a. Structured interview

    b. Unstructured interview

    c. Planned interview

    d. Unplanned interview

108. This type of chart is used to focus attention on any variation in the process and helps the team to determine whether that variation is normal or a result of special circumstances.

    a. Pareto chart

    b. Pie chart

    c. Control chart

    d. Line chart

109. The principal process by which organizations optimize the continuum of care for their patients is:

    a. Utilization management

    b. Services management

    c. Case management

    d. Resource management

110. When the patient's physician contacts a healthcare organization to schedule an episode of care service, the healthcare organization begins which step in the case management process?

    a. Preadmission care planning

    b. Care planning at the time of admission

    c. Review the progress of care

    d. Discharge planning

111. Which of the following is an example of analog data?

    a. CT scan

    b. Photographic, chest x-ray film

    c. MRI exam

    d. EKG tracing

112. The computer-based process of extracting, quantifying, and filtering discrete data that reside in a relational database is called:

    a. Intelligent character recognition

    b. Data mining

    c. Autocoding

    d. Bar coding

113. The primary objective of quality in healthcare for both patient and provider is to:

    a. Keep costs under control

    b. Reduce death rates

    c. Reduce the incidence of infectious diseases

    d. Arrive at the desired outcome

114. Which of the following statements regarding quality management in healthcare is true?

    a. The healthcare industry has exhibited leadership in quality management efforts.

    b. Healthcare quality improvement methods have been adopted from the business sector.

    c. Healthcare quality improvement methods have been adopted from the education sector.

    d. The implementation of quality improvement methods in healthcare has been relatively smooth and seamless.

115. Clinical quality management focuses on the evaluation of:

    a. All healthcare industry processes

    b. Direct care and treatment of patients

    c. Business processes in healthcare

    d. A combination of demographic, financial, and patient care areas

116. Which documents give detailed information about all substances and materials used at a facility, including any hazards associated with them?

    a. Disaster clean-up plan

    b. Hazard vulnerability plan

    c. Material safety data sheets

    d. Substance exposure instruction sheets

117. The Joint Commission has published a list of abbreviations classified as "Do Not Use" for the purpose of:

    a. Assisting coders to read physician handwriting

    b. Preventing potential medication errors due to misinterpretation

    c. Making terminology consistent in preparation for electronic records

    d. Identifying physicians who are dispensing large quantities of drugs

118. Which one of the following is a characteristic of an organized medical staff as recognized by the Joint Commission?

    a. Peer review activities are optional unless requested by a physician.

    b. Fully licensed physicians are permitted by law to provide patient care services.

    c. Delineation of clinical privileges is not necessary.

    d. The medical staff is not subject to medical staff bylaws/rules, regulations, and policies; and is subject to their professional code of ethics.

119. A person who states, "Our main job is to prevent injury and property loss," is primarily concerned with:

    a. Credentialing

    b. Utilization management

    c. Risk management

    d. Severity indexing

120. A database established to identify the level of resource consumption based on clinical evidence is best described as:

    a. Utilization review

    b. Severity index

    c. Risk management

    d. Credentials review

121. Quality improvement focuses on the three performance measures of _____, _____, and _____.

    a. Process, results, mortality

    b. Training, process, results

    c. Structure, process, outcome

    d. Surgery, outcomes, admission

122. The most commonly used data source during quality improvement activities is the:

    a. Health record

    b. Pathology report

    c. Operative index

    d. Patient bills

123. Which of the following items are fundamental parts of a Quality Improvement plan?

    a. Vision, mission, and community outreach

    b. Objectives, values, and performance measures

    c. Values, performance measures, and community outreach

    d. Objective, mission, and accreditation status

124. The government agency that is developing best practice guidelines and working to improve the quality of care in the United States is the:

    a. Institute of Medicine

    b. National Practitioner Data Bank

    c. Agency of Healthcare Research and Quality

    d. Centers for Medicare and Medicaid Services

125. Ultimate responsibility for the quality of care in an acute care organization falls to the:

    a. Safety Committee

    b. Governing body

    c. Centers for Medicare and Medicaid Services

    d. Quality Improvement Steering Committee

126. Performance measures can be described best as:

    a. Methods for data analysis

    b. Safety practices

    c. Statements of expectation

    d. Universal protocols

127. Standardized sets of valid, reliable, and evidence-based measures implemented by the Joint Commission are called:

    a. Sentinel events

    b. Indicator monitoring systems

    c. Core (performance) measures

    d. Technical reporting requirements

128. Blood and blood component usage review, medication usage review, and surgical case review are all examples of:

    a. Activities used in appointing to the medical staff

    b. Medical staff clinical QI activities

    c. Infection control data

    d. Data available through the National Practitioner Data Bank

129. Which of the following are basic functions of the utilization management process?

    a. Preadmission review, claims management, and retrospective review

    b. Discharge planning, review for potentially compensable events, and loss prevention

    c. Discharge planning, retrospective review, and preadmission review

    d. Retrospective review, discharge planning, and review for potentially compensable events

130. The Donabedian Quality Assessment Model includes which three measures?

   a. Plan, do, act

   b. Structure, process, outcome

   c. Indication, process, evaluation

   d. Scope, response, action

131. The process of preventing the spread of communicable diseases in compliance with applicable legal requirements is performed in this quality management function.

   a. Infection control

   b. Clinical quality assessment

   c. Utilization management

   d. Risk management

132. The process of overseeing the medical, legal, and administrative operations within a healthcare organization is performed in this quality management function.

   a. Infection control

   b. Clinical quality management

   c. Utilization management

   d. Risk management

133. The process of determining whether healthcare services meet predetermined standards of care is performed in this quality management function.

   a. Infection control

   b. Clinical quality assessment

   c. Utilization management

   d. Risk management

134. A group of processes used to measure how efficiently healthcare organizations use their resources is performed in what quality management function?

   a. Infection control

   b. Clinical quality assessment

   c. Utilization management

   d. Risk management

135. An assessment of a patient's readiness for placement in a nonacute setting is what function of utilization management?

   a. Admission review

   b. Concurrent review

   c. Discharge planning

   d. Preadmission review

136. This function of the utilization management program determines medical necessity and appropriateness of admission.

    a. Admission review

    b. Concurrent review

    c. Discharge planning

    d. Preadmission review

137. This function of the utilization management program identifies patients who are unsuitable for a particular procedure or admission.

    a. Admission review

    b. Concurrent review

    c. Discharge planning

    d. Preadmission review

138. In this function of the utilization management program, an evaluation occurs at preset intervals to ensure that the patient requires continued care.

    a. Admission review

    b. Concurrent review

    c. Discharge planning

    d. Preadmission review

139. Which of the following are used to report information about mortality and morbidity at local, state, and national levels?

    a. Rates, populations, and ratios

    b. Ratios, proportion, and continuous variables

    c. Proportions, populations, and continuous variables

    d. Proportions, ratios, and rates

140. The following performance standard, "File 50 to 60 records per hour" is an example of a:

    a. Quality standard

    b. Quantity standard

    c. Joint Commission standard

    d. Compliance standard

141. The following performance standard, "Complete five birth certificates per hour" is an example of a:

    a. Quality standard

    b. Quantity standard

    c. Joint Commission standard

    d. Compliance standard

142. The statement "All patients admitted with a diagnosis falling into ICD-9-CM code numbers 800 through 959" represents a possible case definition for what type of registry?

    a. Birth defect registry

    b. Cancer registry

    c. Diabetes registry

    d. Trauma registry

143. A ratio in which *x* is a portion of the whole is called a(n):

    a. Index

    b. Chart

    c. Proportion

    d. Distribution

144. A director of a health information services department plans to do a research project on motivation that involves rewarding some employees for achieving specified goals. A control group will not be rewarded for achieving the same goals. Which entity will need to approve this study?

    a. Institutional review board

    b. Administrative team

    c. Accreditation organization

    d. Medical staff

145. The distribution in this curve is:

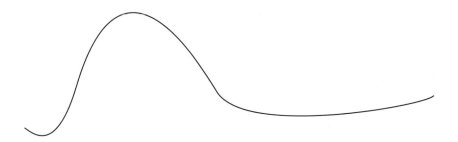

    a. Normal

    b. Bimodal

    c. Skewed left

    d. Skewed right

146. The following table shows the LOS for a sample of 11 discharged patients. Using the data listed, calculate the range.

Patient	Length of Stay
1	1
2	3
3	5
4	3
5	2
6	29
7	3
8	4
9	2
10	1
11	2

  a. 29

  b. 1

  c. 5

  d. 28

147. Community Memorial Hospital discharged nine patients on April 1st. The length of stay for each patient is shown in the following table. What is the median length of stay for this group of patients?

Patient	Number of Days
A	1
B	5
C	3
D	3
E	8
F	8
G	8
H	9
I	9

  a. 5 days

  b. 6 days

  c. 8 days

  d. 9 days

148. Which of the following is true of the median?

    a. It is a measure of variability.

    b. It is difficult to calculate.

    c. It is based on the whole distribution.

    d. It is sensitive to extreme values.

149. The researcher's informed consent form stated that the patients' information would be anonymous. Later, in the application form for IRB approval, the researcher described a coding system to track respondents and nonrespondents. The IRB returned the application to the researcher with the stipulation that the informed consent must be changed. What raised the red flag?

    a. The description of the use of a coding system to track respondents and nonrespondents

    b. The application form for the IRB approval

    c. The researcher's informed consent form

    d. The description of the use of a coding system to track respondents

150. Last year, 73,249 people died from diabetes mellitus in the United States. The total number of deaths from all causes was 2,443,387, and the total population was 288,356,713. Calculate the proportionate mortality ratio for diabetes mellitus.

    a. 0.0003

    b. 10.94

    c. 0.09

    d. 0.03

151. The distribution in this curve is:

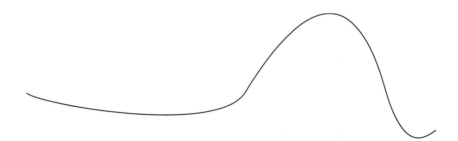

    a. Normal

    b. Bimodal

    c. Skewed left

    d. Skewed right

152. A researcher fails to inform a study participant of the reasonable risks in a study on the effectiveness of a new chemotherapy agent. What ethical principle was violated?

    a. Beneficence

    b. Ethical treatment

    c. Justice

    d. Respect for persons

153. A measure of variability that describes the deviation from the mean of a frequency distribution in the original units of measurement is called the:

    a. Mean

    b. Mode

    c. Standard deviation

    d. Standard variance

154. Which of the following is an external user of hospital data?

    a. Public health department

    b. Medical staff

    c. Hospital administrator

    d. Director of the clinical laboratory

155. You want to graph the average length of stay by sex and service for the month of April. Which graphic tool would you use?

    a. Bar graph

    b. Histogram

    c. Line graph

    d. Pie chart

156. A collection of data that is organized so its contents can easily be accessed, managed, and updated is called a:

    a. Spreadsheet

    b. Database

    c. File

    d. Data table

157. Quality has several components, including appropriateness, technical excellence, _____, and acceptability.

    a. Accuracy of diagnosis

    b. Continuous improvement

    c. Connectivity

    d. Accessibility

158. The generic formula for calculating rate of occurrence is used to calculate hospital-acquired infections in an intensive care unit in a given month. If the number of hospital-acquired infections is the numerator, the denominator would be the:

    a. Number of patients who died of an infection

    b. Number of deaths in the ICU

    c. Number of discharges (including deaths) of ICU patients

    d. Total number of hospital discharges

159. Dr. Jones comes into the HIM department and requests the HIM director to pull all of his records from the previous year in which the principal diagnosis of myocardial infarction was indicated. Where would the HIM director begin to pull these records?

    a. Disease index

    b. Master patient index

    c. Operative index

    d. Physician index

160. In January, Community Hospital had 57 discharges from its Medicine unit. Four patients developed a urinary tract infection while in the hospital. What is the nosocomial infection rate for the Medicine unit for January?

    a. 0.07%

    b. 2.17%

    c. 7%

    d. 217%

161. The practice of quality is most focused on:

    a. Top management

    b. Successful product lines

    c. The customer

    d. Frontline workers

162. All but which of the following are examples of unusual events that healthcare facilities typically must report?

    a. Falls resulting in fractures

    b. Wrong site surgery

    c. Workers' compensation cases

    d. Medical errors

163. Data used to describe a specific health-related population are called:

    a. Reference data

    b. Financial data

    c. Clinical data

    d. Epidemiological data

164. A QI technique that allows groups to narrow the focus of discussion or to make decisions without becoming involved in extended circular discussions is called:

    a. Brainstorming

    b. Benchmarking

    c. Decision-making technique

    d. Nominal group technique

165. According to the Pareto Principle, _____ percent of the sources of a problem are responsible for _____ percent of its actual effects.

    a. 20, 20

    b. 20, 80

    c. 80, 80

    d. 80, 100

166. The most common type of health information is:

    a. Clinical data

    b. Demographic data

    c. Coded data

    d. Epidemiological data

167. This type of data display tool is used to illustrate frequency distributions of continuous variables, such as age or length of stay (LOS).

    a. Bar graph

    b. Histogram

    c. Pie chart

    d. Scatter diagram

Domain III   *Information Technology and Systems*

168. Which of the following is an example of clinical information systems?

    a. Laboratory information system

    b. Staff scheduling system

    c. Patient registration system

    d. Material management system

169. The best reason for implementing IS technology in healthcare is to:

    a. Provide effective and efficient patient care services

    b. Keep up with rapid technological change

    c. Provide a competitive edge in marketing the organization

    d. Support all identified IS initiatives identified by managers in the organization

170. The most common reason given for information system failure is:

    a. Lack of training

    b. No increased benefits gained

    c. Technical failure of hardware and/or software

    d. User resistance

171. To be successful, any information system technology initiative must align with:

    a. Current hardware in use in the facility

    b. The organization's strategic plan

    c. IS department strategies

    d. Health information management initiatives

172. The individual most likely to lead strategic planning for a healthcare organization's information system is the:

    a. CEO

    b. HIM director

    c. CIO

    d. Medical director

173. As a preliminary step in designing an IS strategy, it is important for the steering committee to conduct a scan of the external environment and to:

    a. Build security and privacy constraints

    b. Contact vendors for system bids

    c. Purchase hardware and software components

    d. Conduct an internal environmental assessment

174. An RFP serves two important purposes: it solidifies the planning information and organizational requirements into a single document, and it:

    a. Allows one vendor an advantage over the other potential vendors.

    b. Enables the organization to make decisions quickly.

    c. Provides valuable insights into the vendors operations and products and levels the playing field in terms of asking all the vendors the same questions.

    d. Delineates the organization's system requirements in such a way that a vendor is selected without review of the entire RFP pool.

175. In which phase of the systems development life cycle does initial training on a new information system generally occur?

    a. Analysis

    b. Design

    c. Implementation

    d. Maintenance and evaluation

176. Identifying user information needs is part of the _____ phase of the systems development life cycle.

    a. Analysis

    b. Design

    c. Implementation

    d. Evaluation

177. A key element in effective systems implementation is:

   a. Contract negotiation

   b. User training

   c. System evaluation

   d. RFP analysis

178. An effective tool for implementing a new information system is:

   a. Project management software

   b. Entity relationship diagrams

   c. User documentation

   d. Structured query languages

179. The role of the chief information officer (CIO) focuses on:

   a. Programming applications

   b. Supporting network infrastructure

   c. Installing and maintaining network applications

   d. Strategic information systems planning

180. One strategy for acquiring EHR components from various vendors and interfacing them is:

   a. Best-of-breed

   b. Best-of-fit

   c. Dual core

   d. Integration

181. In which type of health information exchange architectural model does the organization operate much like an application service provider (ASP) or bank vault?

   a. Consolidated

   b. Federated–consistent database

   c. Federated–inconsistent database

   d. Switch

182. Which of the following basic services provided by an HIE organization identifies participating users and systems?

   a. Identity management

   b. Person identification

   c. Registry and directory

   d. Secure data transport

183. A healthcare organization remains committed to purchasing a vendor's product, which the organization finds solid in its financial and administrative applications but weaker in clinical applications. What is the term for this strategy?

    a. Bridge

    b. Best-of-fit

    c. Best-of-breed

    d. Legacy

184. In data capture terminology, data entry as narrative data via keyboarding, dictation, voice recognition, and handwriting recognition is known as:

    a. Free text

    b. A graphical user interface

    c. Natural language processing

    d. Structured data

185. Which of the following basic services provided by an HIE organization matches identifying information to an individual?

    a. Consent management

    b. Person identification

    c. Record locator

    d. Identity management

186. This EHR implementation strategy identifies the sequence of implementing the EHR with regard to various inpatient units, departments, physicians, or other categories of users or sites.

    a. Phased roll-out

    b. Big bang roll-out

    c. Pilot

    d. Straight turnover

187. This EHR turnover strategy continues with its paper processing until the EHR works as planned.

    a. Parallel processing

    b. Phased roll-out

    c. Pilot

    d. Straight turnover

188. This EHR implementation strategy stops its paper processing shortly after the go-live of the system.

    a. Phased roll-out

    b. Big bang roll-out

    c. Pilot

    d. Straight turnover

189. In this EHR implementation strategy virtually every nursing unit, department, clinic, or other organizational unit goes live at the same time with a given component of the EHR.

    a. Phased roll-out

    b. Big bang roll-out

    c. Pilot

    d. Straight turnover

190. Which of the following would likely be recorded on an information systems issues log?

    a. Alan is present every day there is a system test.

    b. Betty reported receiving 25 erroneous e-mail messages.

    c. Dr. Brown effectively uses e-prescribing.

    d. John requested a supply of tamper-proof paper for his office.

191. Protocols that support communication between applications are often referred to as:

    a. Application program

    b. Interface code

    c. Messaging standards

    d. Source code

192. Formatting and/or structuring of captured information that includes the process of analyzing, organizing, and presenting recorded patient information for authentication and inclusion in the patient's healthcare record defines:

    a. Patient health records

    b. Information capture

    c. Report generation

    d. Generating images through x-rays and scans

193. Which organization has created a standard for EHR system functions?

    a. AHIMA

    b. Federal government

    c. HL7

    d. IOM

194. What does *syntax* refer to?

    a. Common meaning of terms in a message

    b. Context of words in narrative form

    c. Structure of data elements in a message

    d. Text processing

195. The process of normalization in a data warehouse works to eliminate:

    a. Access

    b. Redundancy

    c. Transactions

    d. Queries

196. The term used to describe breaking data elements into the level of detail needed to retrieve the data is:

    a. Normalization

    b. Data definitions

    c. Primary key

    d. A database management system

197. A concept that is related to a data warehouse but has a different architecture and tends to undergo more changes is a:

    a. Graphical decision support system

    b. Data marketplace

    c. Snowflake schema

    d. Clinical data repository

198. Which of the following indexes and databases includes patient-identifiable information?

    a. MEDLINE

    b. Clinical trials database

    c. Master patient/population index

    d. UMLS

199. Which of the following is the process of probing and extracting business data and information from a data warehouse and then quantifying and filtering the data for analysis purposes?

    a. Application systems analysis

    b. Multidimensional OLAPs

    c. Data mining

    d. Clinical data repositories

200. A group of computers connected within a relatively small geographic area such as an office building or hospital is what type of network?

    a. Local area network

    b. Wide area network

    c. Wireless local area network

    d. Virtual private network

201. A group of computers that connect across a relatively large geographic distance using telephone or cable services is what type of network?

    a. Local area network

    b. Wide area network

    c. Wireless local area network

    d. Virtual private network

202. A group of devices that connect to a local area network via radio waves is what type of network?

    a. Local area network

    b. Wide area network

    c. Wireless local area network

    d. Virtual private network

203. *Topology* refers to a(n):

    a. Arrangement of a network

    b. Beginning of a network

    c. End point of a network

    d. Network connection

204. What form of logical topology is most widely used today for local area networks?

    a. Bus

    b. Ethernet

    c. Gateway

    d. POTS

205. What is the most commonly used means to transmit data across a wide area network today?

    a. Frame relay

    b. ISDN

    c. POTS

    d. T-lines

206. A transmission medium commonly used to connect portable medical devices to information systems is:

    a. Cable

    b. Infrared light

    c. Microwave

    d. Radio waves

207. In this type of network, all computers on the network receive the same message at the same time, but only one computer at a time can transfer information; and if one segment of the network goes down, the entire network is affected.

    a. Star topology

    b. Ring topology

    c. Bus topology

    d. Logical topology

208. In this type of network configuration, individual computers are connected through a central hub that serves as a traffic cop for the data.

    a. Star topology

    b. Ring topology

    c. Bus topology

    d. Logical topology

209. Which of the following are considered input devices?

    a. Keyboard, printer, and mouse

    b. Touch pad, speech recognition, and printer

    c. Optical character recognition, printer, and mouse

    d. Speech recognition, touch pad, and mouse

210. Mobile input devices are primarily limited in their use by:

    a. Navigational support concerns

    b. Network connectivity support

    c. Portability

    d. Power supply issues

211. Which term is used to describe the device that runs a secondary storage medium?

    a. Central processing unit

    b. Drive

    c. Magnetic disk

    d. Storage network

212. An example of storage technology used to achieve redundancy in the event of a server crash is:

    a. CPU

    b. DVD

    c. RAID

    d. USB

213. Which type of architecture has one powerful central computer that performs all processing and storage functions while sending and receiving data to/from various terminals and printers?

    a. Client/server

    b. Mainframe

    c. Super computer

    d. Web-based

214. The most common architecture used in EHRs in hospitals today is:

    a. Client/server

    b. Mainframe

    c. Network computers

    d. Web-based

215. An important characteristic of web-services architecture is:

a. Freely available software from the web

b. Programs that act as a web browser

c. Use of the Internet for transmission of information

d. Wide area network design

216. HTML and XML are programming languages used to create:

a. Web-enabled applications

b. Expert decision support systems

c. Web browser-based applications

d. Artificial intelligence systems

217. OLAP is the acronym used for:

a. On-time linear analysis program

b. Online linear analytical program

c. Online analytical processing

d. One-time leftover analysis predicament

218. Data mining is a process that involves which of the following?

a. Using reports to measure outcomes

b. Using sophisticated computer technology to sort through an organization's data to identify unusual patterns

c. Producing summary reports for management to run the daily activities of the organization

d. Producing detailed reports to track productivity

219. This data mining technique discovers relationships between attributes within data sets and displays them in a linked network graph to enable the user to better visualize the patterns.

a. Machine learning

b. Linkage analysis

c. Neural networks

d. Logistic regression

220. By querying the organizational data, you find that patients admitted on a weekend have a mean length of stay that is 1.3 days longer than patients who are admitted Monday through Friday. This method of finding information is called:

a. Structuring query language

b. Data mining

c. Multidimensional data structuring

d. Satisficing

221. What must be in place to enhance the retrieval process for scanned documents?

    a. Electronic signature

    b. Indexing system

    c. RFID device

    d. Table of contents

222. Which of the following stores a clinical image in a computer?

    a. CDA

    b. FDA

    c. PACS

    d. XML

223. In which record numbering system is the patient assigned a health record number on the first visit that is kept for all subsequent visits?

    a. Unit numbering

    b. Index unit numbering

    c. Serial-unit numbering

    d. Serial numbering

224. Which numerical filing system results in an even distribution of records and ensures activity throughout the filing area?

    a. Serial-unit filing system

    b. Serial filing system

    c. Unit filing system

    d. Terminal-digit filing system

225. What is an advantage of the unit filing system?

    a. All records for a specific patient, both inpatient and outpatient, are filed together.

    b. The charts have to be split into volumes for filing.

    c. The hospital can accommodate a large outpatient clinic with many return visits.

    d. Joint Commission approval is automatic because all parts of the record are filed together.

226. Which microfilming system is best when you plan to file the film using a terminal-digit unit record system?

    a. Jackets

    b. Roll

    c. Cartridge

    d. Rotary

227. For an EHR to provide robust clinical decision support, what critical element must be present?

    a. Structured data

    b. Internet connection

    c. Physician portal

    d. Standard vocabulary

228. Which of the following is a concept designed to help standardize clinical content for sharing between providers?

    a. Continuity of care record

    b. Interoperability

    c. Personal health record

    d. SNOMED

229. In addition to bar codes on health record documents, what other forms of recognition characteristics enhance the accuracy of forms indexing features?

    a. Access controls

    b. COLD

    c. OCR

    d. Workflow

230. Review of disease indexes, pathology reports, and radiation therapy reports is part of which function in the cancer registry?

    a. Case definition

    b. Case finding

    c. Follow-up

    d. Reporting

231. Which of the following is a database from the National Health Care Survey that uses the health record as a data source?

    a. National Health Provider Inventory

    b. National Ambulatory Medical Care Survey

    c. National Employer Health Insurance Survey

    d. National Infectious Disease Inventory

232. A protocol to pass data from the R-ADT system of one vendor to the laboratory information system of another vendor is called:

    a. OLAP

    b. Integration

    c. TCP/IP

    d. Interface

233. Which of the following statements is true of structured query language (SQL)?

    a. It is both a data manipulation and data back-up mechanism.

    b. It defines data elements and manipulates and controls data.

    c. It is the computer language associated with document imaging.

    d. Users are not able to query a relational database.

234. Which of the following is a kind of technology that focuses on data security?

    a. Clinical decision support

    b. Bit-mapped data

    c. Firewalls

    d. Smart cards

235. The basic component of a(n) _____ is an object that contains both data and their relationships in a single structure.

    a. Object-oriented database

    b. Relational database

    c. Access database

    d. Structured database

236. Copying data onto tapes and storing the tapes at a distant location is an example of:

    a. Data backup

    b. Data mapping

    c. Data recovery

    d. Data storage for recovery

237. Ensuring that data have been accessed or modified only by those authorized to do so is a function of:

    a. Data integrity

    b. Data quality

    c. Data granularity

    d. Logging functions

238. In Medical Center Hospital's clinical information system, nurses may write nursing notes and may read all parts of the patient health record for patients on the unit in which they work. This type of authorized use is called:

    a. Password limitation

    b. Security clearance

    c. Access privilege assignment

    d. User grouping

239. Which of the following controls external access to a network?

    a. Access controls

    b. Alarms

    c. Encryption

    d. Firewall

Practice Questions

240. Data edits included in software to detect errors are used to check the _____ of the data.

   a. Validity
   b. Reliability
   c. Timeliness
   d. Compatibility

241. Passwords provide:

   a. Access control
   b. Data authentication
   c. Entity authentication
   d. Firewall control

242. Identifying appropriate users of specific information is a function of:

   a. Access control
   b. Nosology
   c. Data modeling
   d. Workflow modeling

243. Authorization management involves:

   a. The process used to protect the reliability of a database
   b. Limiting user access to a database
   c. Allowing unlimited use of the database
   d. Developing definitions for database elements

244. The security devices situated between the routers of a private network and a public network to protect the private network from unauthorized users are called:

   a. Audit trails
   b. Passwords
   c. Firewalls
   d. Encryptors

245. Which of the following is an example of an e-health application?

   a. Bedside nursing care
   b. Appointment scheduling
   c. Direct patient care
   d. Emergency care records

246. A single point of personalized web access through which to find and deliver information, applications, and services is called a(n):

   a. Keyhole
   b. Entry way
   c. WWW
   d. Portal

247. The process of integrating healthcare facility systems requires the creation of:

    a. Data warehouses

    b. E-health initiatives

    c. Enterprise master patient indexes

    d. Electronic data interchange

248. In today's healthcare organization, physicians use the _____ to access multiple sources of patient information within the organization's network.

    a. Data repository

    b. Clinical information system

    c. Data warehouse

    d. Clinician portal

249. A drug interaction alert would be a typical function of a:

    a. Data warehouse

    b. Data repository

    c. Data mart

    d. Clinical decision support system

250. When a physician practice has a high revisit rate and an EHR that supports discrete data entry, the best data conversion strategy is:

    a. Abstracting

    b. Document imaging

    c. Interfacing

    d. Filing paper charts

251. Mobile professionals in a hospital are most likely to use which form of human-computer interface?

    a. Computer on wheels

    b. Desktop computer

    c. Personal digital assistant

    d. Terminal

252. A certain system gathers data from a variety of sources and assists in providing structure to the data using various analytical models and visual tools in order to facilitate and improve the ultimate outcome in decision-making tasks associated with nonroutine and nonrepetitive problems. What is this type of system called?

    a. Decision support system

    b. Health information system

    c. Six-Sigma system

    d. Electronic patient record system

253. Which reasoning element is usually referred to in a knowledge-based DSS?

    a. A database

    b. A gathering place

    c. A GUI

    d. An inference engine

254. Community Hospital just added a new system that changed the way data move throughout the facility. Which of the following would need to be updated to reflect this change?

    a. Data dictionary

    b. Entity relationship diagram

    c. Data flow diagram

    d. Semantic object model

255. An evaluation of the benefits that have accrued from the EHR investment that is performed at specific milestones in the life of the project and used to help in future systems planning, designing, and implementing is called:

    a. Benefits realization study

    b. Goal setting exercise

    c. Cost-benefit feasibility study

    d. Productivity improvement study

256. Community Hospital has a database that is used by many different systems and has real-time data. This is an example of a:

    a. Data warehouse

    b. Data mart

    c. Data repository

    d. Data model

257. Electronic document management system (EDMS) would enable which of the following changes to occur in an HIM department?

    a. Change record retention schedule to one year

    b. Eliminate transcription

    c. Reduce coding errors

    d. Shift release of information to point of service

258. A key element in the structure of a decision support system (DSS) that assists in presenting the results to the user is called the:

    a. Brain of the DSS

    b. Graphical user interface

    c. Inference engine

    d. Knowledge base

259. Standardizing medical terminology to avoid differences in naming various medical conditions and procedures (such as the synonyms bunionectomy, McBride procedure, and repair of hallus valgus) is one purpose of:

    a. Transaction standards

    b. Content and structure standards

    c. Vocabulary standards

    d. Security standards

260. A critical early step in designing an EHR in which the characteristics of each data element are defined is to develop a(n):

    a. Accreditation manual

    b. Core content

    c. Continuity of care record

    d. Data dictionary

261. To be successful, a regional health information network is dependent on:

    a. Stakeholder consensus on local regional needs

    b. Federal funding

    c. Enabling legislation by the state

    d. Fees paid by consumers

Domain IV *Organization and Management*

262. A leader solicits input from team members by going from one to the next around the table or room and each team member comments on the issue in turn or passes until the next round, and this process continues until participants have no new ideas to suggest or until the time period set in the meeting's agenda has elapsed. This activity is an example of:

    a. Benchmarking

    b. Decision-making technique

    c. Structured brainstorming

    d. Unstructured brainstorming

263. This predefined process icon [ ] is used in flowcharting to indicate:

    a. A process when actions are being performed by humans

    b. A point in the process at which participants must evaluate the status of the process

    c. Formal procedures that participants are expected to carry out the same way every time

    d. A point in the process where the participants must record data in paper-based or computer-based formats

264. This manual input icon ⬜ is used in flowcharting to indicate:

    a. A process when actions are being performed by a computer

    b. A point in the process at which participants must evaluate the status of the process

    c. Formal procedures that participants are expected to carry out the same way every time

    d. A point in the process where the participants must record data in paper-based or computer-based formats

265. An idea-generation technique in which a team leader solicits creative input from team members is called:

    a. Benchmarking

    b. Systematic input

    c. Brainstorming

    d. Team input

266. A graphic tool used to organize and prioritize ideas after a brainstorming session is called a(n):

    a. Affinity diagram

    b. Cause-and-effect diagram

    c. Brainstorming diagram

    d. Sentinel diagram

267. Which of the following elements is found in a charge description master?

    a. ICD-9-CM code

    b. Procedure or service charge

    c. Patient disposition

    d. Procedural service date

268. A kinesthetic learner prefers to learn by:

    a. Hearing

    b. Reading

    c. Watching

    d. Practicing

269. The most common form of e-learning delivery is:

    a. Asynchronous web-based

    b. Synchronous web-based

    c. CD-ROM/DVD-ROM

    d. M-learning

270. Which of the following are the traditional four managerial functions?

    a. Leading, negotiating, planning, and operations management

    b. Controlling, planning, operations management, and management by objectives

    c. Leading, controlling, organizing, and planning

    d. Planning, negotiating, controlling, and leading

271. The span of management refers to the:

    a. Number of roles a manager performs

    b. Number of subordinates a manager supervises

    c. Ratio of managers to workers in an organization

    d. Diversity of the range of products or services

272. What actions might be taken to reduce the risks of groupthink?

    a. High cohesion without interaction with outside groups

    b. Monitoring the degree of consensus and disagreement

    c. The leader states his or her opinion early to influence the rest of the group

    d. Limit organizational controls

273. Feedback is most useful when:

    a. A great amount is provided at one time.

    b. The person receiving it requests it.

    c. It is collected and presented at the end of the year.

    d. When it focuses on the value of the person rather than the behavior.

274. Which of the following are alternate work scheduling techniques?

    a. Compressed workweek, open systems, and job sharing

    b. Flextime, telecommuting, and compressed workweek

    c. Telecommuting, open systems, and flextime

    d. Flextime, outsourcing, compressed workweek

275. The statement "Enter birth date using the format MMDDYYYY" would most likely be found in a:

    a. Job procedure

    b. Work distribution chart

    c. Workflow process

    d. Movement diagram

276. In setting up systems to measure work performance, it is critical to establish:

    a. Aesthetics

    b. Standards

    c. Movement diagrams

    d. Work distribution charts

277. An organization's standards should reflect its:

    a. Goals

    b. Vision

    c. Procedures

    d. Affinity groupings

278. The statement "Coding of inpatient records must be completed at a 98 percent accuracy rate" is an example of a:

    a. Goal

    b. Vision statement

    c. Qualitative standard

    d. Quantitative standard

279. Which of the following would be considered discriminatory practices in the employment setting?

    a. Denial of employment based on criminal record

    b. Screening out an applicant that does not meet the minimum qualifications for the position

    c. Denial of employment based on religion

    d. Hiring a person based on vision of the organization

280. Under the Americans with Disabilities Act, employees receive protection with respect to their job duties if they are able to perform the necessary functions of a job:

    a. As the job exists

    b. With reasonable accommodations

    c. With changes to the work arrangements

    d. While sharing the job with another employee

281. Collective bargaining refers to:

    a. Salary negotiations between managers and administration

    b. Hearings to establish whether sexual harassment occurred in the workplace

    c. Contract negotiations between a union and an employer

    d. Hearings to negotiate salaries

282. What law requires employers to create a safe work environment and comply with health standards?

    a. FLSA

    b. NLRA

    c. ERISA

    d. OSHA

283. The financial statement that communicates the financial position of an organization at a certain point in time is called the:

    a. Income statement

    b. Balance sheet

    c. Statement of cash flows

    d. Statement of retained earnings

284. The financial statement that presents a statement of operations by showing revenue and expenses over a period of time is called the:

    a. Income statement

    b. Balance sheet

    c. Statement of cash flows

    d. Statement of retained earnings

285. All variances (as related to accounting) should be labeled as either:

    a. Good or bad

    b. Favorable or unfavorable

    c. Positive or negative

    d. Over budget or under budget

286. Capital budgeting differs from operational budgeting in what manner?

    a. It is generally limited to one fiscal year.

    b. It involves high dollar purchases and multiple year projects.

    c. It is usually started after completing the operating budget.

    d. It is for purchases other than equipment.

287. In accounting, the "matching" principle means:

    a. The accounts of an entity should be kept separate from the personal transactions of its owners.

    b. Expenses should be reported in the same period as the revenues they helped produce.

    c. Assets should be reported at their historic cost.

    d. Accountants should not overstate liabilities or expenses when making an estimate.

288. Which of the following lists are all assets accounts?

    a. Cash, accounts receivable, and salaries

    b. Buildings, inventory, and accounts payable

    c. Equipment, accounts receivable, and revenue

    d. Cash, accounts receivable, and savings

289. A purchase order ensures that the item purchased:

    a. Meets functional requirements

    b. Has been properly authorized for purchase

    c. Will be shipped immediately

    d. Is warranted for a least a year

290. The GAAP and GAAS standards for accounting and auditing are established by the:

    a. Center for Medicare and Medicaid Services

    b. Health Care Financing Administration

    c. Security and Exchange Commission

    d. Financial Accounting Standards Board

291. Net income is defined as the:

   a. Difference between revenue and expenses

   b. Difference between total assets and total liabilities

   c. Difference between revenue and total liabilities

   d. Difference between net assets and expenses

292. Which financial statement reflects the extent to which an organization's revenues exceed its expenses?

   a. Balance sheet

   b. Statement of cash flow

   c. Statement of retained earnings

   d. Income statement

293. Blackduck Hospital has a fiscal year that ends on September 30. For this hospital, the third quarter ends on:

   a. June 30

   b. March 31

   c. December 31

   d. August 31

294. Services rendered and billed to customers for future payment create transactions that are posted to:

   a. Accounts payable and revenue

   b. Accounts receivable and cash

   c. Accounts payable and accounts receivable

   d. Accounts receivable and revenue

295. What basic accounting principle requires that organizations follow the same accounting rules from year to year?

   a. Disclosure

   b. Reliability

   c. Matching

   d. Consistency

296. An analysis of a company's liquidity attempts to measure the company's ability to:

   a. Meet long-term debt payments

   b. Pay dividends each year

   c. Meet current debt payments

   d. Make a profit

297. Which of the following is an example of a 501(c)(3) organization?

   a. Hospital Corporation of America

   b. American Health Information Management Association

   c. American Cancer Society

   d. Blue Cross/Blue Shield

298. Determining costs associated with EHR hardware and software acquisition, implementation, and ongoing maintenance represents which type of analysis?

    a. Benefits realization study

    b. Goal setting exercise

    c. Cost-benefit feasibility study

    d. Productivity improvement study

299. Which of the following describes task structure?

    a. How much authority the leader has to direct others

    b. How different workers' styles interact in completing the task

    c. How clearly and how well the task goal, procedures, and common solutions are defined

    d. What steps to take to reward staff

300. A leader whose personal style instills loyalty and commitment and inspires people to perform beyond expectations toward a vision would be best described as:

    a. Transactional

    b. Normative

    c. Charismatic

    d. Inventive

301. A leader effectively using Leader-Member Exchange theory would be viewed by the "out group" as:

    a. Showing unfair preference to personally favorite employees

    b. Being fair to the out-group

    c. Requiring too much effort from the out-group for too few benefits

    d. Requiring too much extra work from the in-group

302. Which of the following statements is most accurate regarding the difference between leaders and managers?

    a. Managers strive for change while leaders promote efficiency.

    b. Managers ask how something should be done and leaders ask why.

    c. Leaders attend to danger and uncertainty, while managers seek out opportunity in them.

    d. Leaders use analytic thinking while managers use more flexible thinking styles.

303. In management theory, the Peter Principle refers to the:

    a. Leadership findings of Peters and Waterman's study on excellence

    b. Belief that people are promoted to their level of incompetency

    c. Belief that most successful leaders have excellent communication skills

    d. Belief that leader intuition is generally more accurate than knowledge

304. Systems' thinking focuses on understanding of which of the following?

    a. The relationships among parts and processes of the organization and how they work together

    b. The operational level of strategy

    c. How successful leader traits develop and may be overused

    d. The formulation of envisioning used by the leader to develop esprit

305. Which of the following best categorizes the group of adopters who comprise the backbone of the organization, are conventional and deliberate in their decisions, and form a bridge with other adopter categories?

    a. Innovators

    b. Early adopters

    c. Early majority

    d. Late majority

306. Laggard adopters best serve the function of:

    a. Providing a group for downsizing the organization

    b. Providing vision for the organization

    c. Seeking reasons to innovate

    d. Keeping the organization from changing too fast

307. During the early stages of diffusion, there is a shorter period between becoming aware of an innovation and adopting it. The best description of the innovation adoption shown by a line is which of the following:

    a. Straight-line showing gradual increase

    b. J-shaped curve

    c. S-shaped curve

    d. D-shaped curve

308. Which of the following statements most accurately describes management fads?

    a. They are inaccurate, mistaken, and offer little to organizations.

    b. Extensive use of fads tends to motivate workers.

    c. Fads often have useful aspects to them.

    d. Fads nearly always fail to perform and should be dismissed.

309. The goal of organizational development (OD) practitioners is to:

    a. Be continually available to the organization over many years

    b. Diagnose the organization for the administration

    c. Make strong and clear recommendations about what an organization should do

    d. Engage the organization in understanding itself

310. Which of the following represent the stages of reflective learning?

    a. Doing, reflection, interpretation, application

    b. Feeling, thinking, doing

    c. Analysis, antithesis, synthesis

    d. Synthesizing, doing, analyzing, reflecting

311. What kind of planning addresses long-term needs and sets comprehensive plans of action?

    a. Tactical

    b. Operational

    c. Strategic

    d. Administrative

312. When an effective leader provides employees with information, responsibility, authority, and trust, this is called:

    a. Empowerment

    b. Promotion

    c. Vision

    d. Delegation

313. What best describes servant leadership?

    a. Staying with one's vision despite daily realities

    b. Using coercion to build consensus

    c. Focusing on the greatest good for the larger society

    d. Assuming people are up to no good regardless of their behaviors

314. Which of the following statements describes a critical skill for a strategic manager?

    a. Ability to change direction quickly

    b. Ability to deliver results on budget

    c. Ability to envision relationships between trends and opportunities

    d. Ability to design jobs and match peoples' skill to them

315. The concept of organizational learning is the centerpiece of:

    a. Tichy's systems approach

    b. Kotter's model for leading change

    c. Kaplan's strategy maps

    d. Kolb's Learning Loop

316. Successful strategic managers understand that three competencies are common to all successful change and that these competencies can and must be developed. These three are:

    a. Leadership, change management, and strategic development

    b. Organizational learning, visioning, and leadership

    c. Visioning, managing, and change management

    d. Improvement, visioning, and managing

317. The process by which an organization gets to its future state or its vision for improved processes is known as:

    a. Change management

    b. Strategic planning

    c. Tactical planning

    d. Vision and mission statements

318. Which work measurement tool uses random sample observations to obtain information about the performance of an entire department?

    a. Performance measurement

    b. Work distribution

    c. Work sampling

    d. Performance controls

319. Non-self-correcting controls are also known as _____ controls.

    a. Preventive

    b. Feedback

    c. Performance

    d. Sampling

320. Which of the following statements about customer service is true?

    a. All customers are internal.

    b. Employees do not fit the definition of customer.

    c. Customers are the reason for the collective work of an organization.

    d. It is not important to get customer feedback if the organization is meeting its mission.

321. In a flow process chart, the information presented in a circle represents a(n):

    a. Inspection

    b. Operation

    c. Delay

    d. Archiving function

322. Which of the following factors is a consideration when revising a project to keep it on track?

    a. Adding an additional required feature

    b. Adding a person to help another project team member

    c. Holding a kickoff meeting

    d. Not allowing overtime

323. In project management, what is risk?

    a. An answer to an unknown question

    b. A situation that can affect the success of the project

    c. A situation that prevents completion of a project task

    d. A change in the project scope

324. In project management, what is a baseline?

    a. Documentation of the project issues

    b. Project definition document

    c. Original estimates for the work effort, cost, and project time line

    d. Tracking of project progress

325. Which of the following are attributes of both projects and daily operations?

    a. Defined start dates

    b. Roles and responsibilities

    c. Set budget or cost

    d. Defined finish dates

326. The project management life cycle includes which of the following activities?

    a. System selection

    b. Conducting a variance analysis

    c. Securing approval for the project

    d. Formulating a project office

327. Which of the following is a type of project team structure discussed in the project management literature?

    a. Tree

    b. Dynamic

    c. Quantitative

    d. Matrixed

328. In project management, what is a work breakdown structure?

    a. List of the project deliverables

    b. Hierarchical list of the project tasks

    c. Document that defines team roles and responsibilities

    d. List of project scope changes

329. In project management, what is a project scope?

    a. Project budget

    b. Magnitude of the work to be done

    c. Project schedule

    d. Quality of the work products

330. Which organizational unit(s) is (are) responsible for defining project management procedures and best practices?

   a. Stakeholders

   b. Project office

   c. Project resources

   d. Steering committee

331. What is the purpose of the project charter or statement of work in project management?

   a. Detail the tasks to be performed

   b. Set expectations for the what, when, and how of the project

   c. Document project issues

   d. Provide detail estimates for work effort and start and finish dates

332. Which of the following is a type of project communication?

   a. Establish change control

   b. Status reports

   c. Department organization chart

   d. Celebrating success

333. The people or groups of people in an organization who will be affected by a project are the project's:

   a. Sponsors

   b. Stakeholders

   c. Managers

   d. Resources

334. The critical path for a project determines its:

   a. Task sequence

   b. Deliverables

   c. Dependencies

   d. Duration

335. Which of the following is true concerning an EHR project manager?

   a. Most commonly chairs the EHR steering committee

   b. Must demonstrate leadership skills

   c. Not a member of the EHR steering committee

   d. Plays an inactive role on the EHR steering committee

336. In the following figure, identify the component of the project plan labeled as C.

A				1/12	1/13	1/14	1/15	1/16	1/19	1/20
1.	🗎	1. Test ADT-Lab interface		C						
2.		1.1 Write test scenario	Dr. Smith							
					D		E			
3.	✓	1.2 Load test data	John							
	B									
4.		1.3 Execute lab order	Mary							

    a. Duration of major task

    b. Task completed

    c. Task progress

    d. Dependency

337. In the following figure, identify the component of the project plan labeled as D.

A				1/12	1/13	1/14	1/15	1/16	1/19	1/20
1.	🗎	1. Test ADT-Lab interface		C						
2.		1.1 Write test scenario	Dr. Smith							
					D		E			
3.	✓	1.2 Load test data	John							
	B									
4.		1.3 Execute lab order	Mary							

    a. Row numbers

    b. Task completed

    c. Task progress

    d. Dependency

338. The accounting term for a cost that when expressed on a per unit basis will remain constant over a change of volumes is:

    a. Variable

    b. Indirect

    c. Fixed

    d. Direct

339. The accounting term for a cost that *cannot* be economically traced to a product or service is:

    a. Liability

    b. Indirect

    c. Fixed

    d. Equity

340. The accounting term for a cost that will vary with changes in volumes or units of production is:

    a. Variable

    b. Indirect

    c. Fixed

    d. Direct

341. The accounting term for a cost that can be traced to a specific service or product is:

    a. Variable

    b. Indirect

    c. Fixed

    d. Direct

342. Which of the following departments are responsible for revenue cycle management in a hospital?

    a. Volunteer services, admitting, and housekeeping

    b. Patient financial services, health information management, and admitting

    c. Admitting, food services, and accounting

    d. Health information management, billing, and volunteer services

343. Which of the following is used to reconcile accounts in the patient accounting department?

    a. Explanation of benefits

    b. Medicare code editor

    c. Preauthorization form

    d. Fee schedule

344. In a typical acute-care setting, Admitting is located in which revenue cycle area?

    a. Pre-claims submission

    b. Claims processing

    c. Accounts receivable

    d. Claims reconciliation/collections

345. In a typical acute-care setting, Aging of Accounts reports are monitored in which revenue cycle area?

    a. Pre-claims submission

    b. Claims processing

    c. Accounts receivable

    d. Claims reconciliation/collections

346. In a typical acute-care setting, Charge Capture is located in which revenue cycle area?

    a. Pre-claims submission

    b. Claims processing

    c. Accounts receivable

    d. Claims reconciliation/collections

347. In a typical acute-care setting, Patient Education of Payment Policies is located in which revenue cycle area?

    a. Pre-claims submission

    b. Claims processing

    c. Accounts receivable

    d. Claims reconciliation and collections

348. In a typical acute-care setting, the Explanation of Benefits, Medicare Summary Notice, and Remittance Advice documents (provided by the payer) are monitored in which revenue cycle area?

    a. Pre-claims submission

    b. Claims processing

    c. Accounts receivable

    d. Claims reconciliation and collections

349. In a typical acute-care setting, which revenue cycle area uses an internal auditing system (scrubber) to ensure error-free claims (clean claims) are submitted to third-party payers?

    a. Pre-claims submission

    b. Claims processing

    c. Accounts receivable

    d. Claims reconciliation and collections

350. Dr. Jones dies while still in active medical practice. He leaves incomplete records at Medical Center Hospital. The best way for the HIM department to handle these incomplete records is to:

    a. Have the administrator of the hospital complete them.

    b. Have the charge nurse on the respective nursing units complete them.

    c. Ask the chief of staff to complete them.

    d. File the incomplete records with a notation about the physician's death.

351. The Act that places controls on labor unions and the relationships between unions and their member is:

    a. Fair Labor Standards Act

    b. Labor-Management Reporting and Disclosure Act

    c. Union Control Act

    d. Workers' Adjustment Retraining and Notification Act

352. The Act that prohibits age-based employment discrimination against individuals between 40 and 70 years of age is:

    a. Equal Pay Act of 1963

    b. Age Discrimination in Employment Act

    c. Taft-Hartley Act

    d. Family and Medical Leave Act

353. The Act that addresses wage disparities based on sex is:

    a. Age Discrimination in Employment Act

    b. Labor Management Relations Act

    c. National Pay Parity Act of 1987

    d. Equal Pay Act of 1963

354. The Act designed to afford protection to disabled employees is:

    a. Americans with Disabilities Act of 1990

    b. Civil Rights Act of 1964

    c. Equal Pay Act of 1963

    d. National Pay Parity Act of 1987

355. The Act that provides for the development and enforcement of standards for health and safety at work is:

    a. Rehabilitation Act of 1973

    b. Occupational Safety and Health Act

    c. National Labor Relations Act

    d. Americans with Disability Act

356. The Act that establishes minimum wages and maximum hours of employment is called the:

    a. Equal Pay Act

    b. Civil Rights Act

    c. Fair Labor Standards Act

    d. National Labor Relations Act

357. Laws that give an employee a legal way to receive compensation for injuries on the job are:

    a. Rehabilitation

    b. Workers' compensation

    c. Equal pay

    d. Fair labor

358. A physician who provides care in a healthcare facility, is not employed by the facility and therefore not under the direct control or supervision of another, and is personally responsible for his or her negligent acts and carries his or her own professional liability insurance is considered a(n) _____ to the healthcare facility.

    a. Agent

    b. Independent contractor

    c. Supervisor

    d. Vendor

359. Generally, substantial performance by one party to a contract will obligate the other party:

    a. To perform their contractual obligations

    b. Not to perform their contractual obligations

    c. To void the contract

    d. To invalidate the contract

360. For a contract to be valid, it must include three elements. Which of the following is one of those elements?

    a. Assumption of risk

    b. Consideration

    c. Statue of limitations

    d. Proposal

361. The Act that prohibits private employers and state and local governments from discriminating on the basis of race, color, religion, sex, or national origin is:

    a. Americans with Disability Act

    b. Civil Rights Act of 1964

    c. Equal Pay Act

    d. Rehabilitation Act of 1973

362. Placing a condition about the award of a contract for laboratory services on the provision of an "under the table" percentage payback to a physician who has the ability to influence the decision on who is awarded the contract is called a(n):

    a. Arbitration

    b. Criminal bribery

    c. Kickback

    d. Solicitation

363. A pharmacist who submits Medicaid claims for reimbursement on brand name drugs when less expensive generic drugs were actually dispensed has committed the crime of:

    a. Criminal negligence

    b. Fraud

    c. Perjury

    d. Products' liability

364. This Act allows employees to be granted a leave of absence for a variety of reasons, including personal or family illness, pregnancy, or military service.

    a. Age Discrimination in Employment Act

    b. Equal Pay Act of 1963

    c. Family and Medical Leave Act

    d. Taft-Hartley Act

365. Which of the following techniques is useful in educating adults?

   a. Criticism

   b. Disregard for their learning needs

   c. Reinforcement

   d. Setting exceptionally high standards

366. Which of the following is considered a viable solution to a staff recruitment problem for coding and transcription shortages?

   a. Delegation

   b. Job distribution

   c. Overtime

   d. Telecommuting

367. What is the best method to use in training a large number of employees in the same location on largely factual knowledge?

   a. Classroom lecture

   b. Web-based chat rooms

   c. Teleconferencing

   d. CD-ROM

368. Annual renewal of fire safety and disaster preparedness are topics that may be addressed best through training known as:

   a. Job rotation

   b. Customer service

   c. In-service education

   d. Pay for performance

369. When an encoding system was installed at Community Memorial Hospital, coders initially found the new system overwhelming and were frustrated because their productivity decreased significantly. This experience represents the first stages of a(n):

   a. Incentive system

   b. Flex system

   c. In-service program

   d. Learning curve

370. Which of the following is an element of the external environment that should be part of a manager's routine scanning?

   a. The opinions of administration

   b. The opinions of employees

   c. Changes in healthcare policy and regulation

   d. What is happening in other departments within the organization

371. Which of the following commonly known examples from business best illustrates a failure of management to do effective environmental scanning?

    a. Enron's collapse

    b. Devaluation of "dotcom" stocks

    c. IBM's slow entry into the PC market

    d. Coca Cola's release and then retraction of "new" Coke from the market

372. A strategy map can be a useful tool because it:

    a. Provides a record of progress toward goals

    b. Provides a visual framework for integrating strategies

    c. Enables others to better understand the vision underlying change

    d. Enables assigning essential resources to executing the plan

373. According to Kotter, creating a sense of urgency is critical to successful change. What example best illustrates an effective technique for creating a sense of urgency by minimizing sources of complacency?

    a. Laying out the vision and informing employees that their jobs are at stake

    b. Convening a project steering committee to expand ownership of the vision and agenda

    c. Bringing in a consultant to design the vision and message

    d. Completing a detailed plan and then engaging staff to carry out the implementation

374. Which of the following is a recommended approach for quick-starting change programs?

    a. Convening nominal groups

    b. Rapid prototyping

    c. Researching alternatives

    d. Surveying other HIM department managers

375. Training provided at the point where it is most useful is called:

    a. Just-in-time training

    b. Sensory training

    c. Simulation

    d. Incentive

376. Which tool is used to determine the most critical areas for training and education for a group of employees?

    a. Performance evaluation

    b. Needs assessment

    c. Orientation assessment

    d. Job specification

377. What is the best way to evaluate how much an employee learns from on-the-job training?

   a. Performance evaluation

   b. Competency assessment

   c. Annual review

   d. Exit interview

378. The least effective incentive for reducing employee turnover is:

   a. Automatic annual pay increase not tied to performance

   b. Pay increase based on both individual and team goal achievement

   c. Pay increase based on quality as well as quantity of work produced

   d. Individual reward to be selected from website

379. The primary goal of organization-sponsored learning is to help employees:

   a. Remain motivated and loyal

   b. Develop effective work habits

   c. Develop managerial skills

   d. Position themselves for career advancement

380. Joe is hired as a floater in a health information department to fill in wherever help is needed. He learns the jobs of several employees. This is an example of:

   a. Outsourcing

   b. Physical training

   c. Cross training

   d. Performance evaluation

381. Heather and Jim are both coders at Medical Center Hospital. The hospital allows them to set their own hours as long as one of them is in the office between 9:00 a.m. and 3:00 p.m. so they are accessible to physicians. This kind of work arrangement is called:

   a. Telecommuting

   b. Compressed workweek

   c. Outsourcing

   d. Flex time

382. Employers should provide jobs with which of the following characteristics in order to retain today's workers?

   a. Predictability

   b. Creativity

   c. Stability

   d. Automatic pay for length of service

Domain V *Privacy, Security, and Confidentiality*

383. Under the HIPAA Security Rule, these types of safeguards have to do with protecting the environment:

    a. Administrative

    b. Physical

    c. Security

    d. Technical

384. What is the legal term used to define the protection of health information in a patient–provider relationship?

    a. Access

    b. Confidentiality

    c. Privacy

    d. Security

385. One of the four general requirements a covered entity must adhere to in order to be in compliance with the HIPAA Security Rule includes the following:

    a. Ensure the confidentiality, integrity, and addressability of ePHI

    b. Ensure the confidentiality, integrity, and accuracy of ePHI

    c. Ensure the confidentiality, integrity, and availability of ePHI

    d. Ensure the confidentiality, integrity, and accountability of ePHI

386. The Uniform Health Care Decisions Act ranks the next-of-kin in the following order for medical decision-making purposes:

    a. Adult sibling; adult child; spouse; parent

    b. Parent; spouse; adult child; adult sibling

    c. Spouse; parent; adult sibling; adult child

    d. Spouse; adult child; parent; adult sibling

387. Health Insurance Portability and Accountability Act's Privacy Rule states that "_____ used for the purposes of treatment, payment, or healthcare operations does not require patient authorization to allow providers access, use, or disclosure." However, only the _____ information needed to satisfy the specified purpose can be used or disclosed.

    a. Demographic information; minimum necessary

    b. Protected health information; minimum necessary

    c. Protected health information; diagnostic

    d. Demographic information; diagnostic

388. Which of the following is a direct command that requires an individual or a representative of an organization to appear in court or to present an object to the court?

    a. Judicial decision

    b. Subpoena

    c. Credential

    d. Regulation

389. A patient having an adverse reaction to a drug correctly administered would be an example of which type of tort liability?

    a. Intentional

    b. Unintentional negligence

    c. Strict liability

    d. Institutional liability

390. The age of majority in most states is:

    a. 16 and older

    b. 17 and older

    c. 18 and older

    d. 21 and older

391. Mary Jones has been declared legally incompetent by the court. Mrs. Jones' sister has been appointed her legal guardian. Her sister is requesting a copy of Mrs. Jones' health records. Of the options listed here, what is the best course of action?

    a. Comply with the sister's request but first request documentation from the sister that she is Mary Jones' legal guardian

    b. Provide the information as requested by the sister

    c. Require that Mary Jones authorize the release of her health information to the sister

    d. Refer the sister to Mary Jones' doctor

392. A competent adult female has a diagnosis of ovarian cancer and while on the operating table suffers a stroke and is in a coma. Her son would like to access her health records from a clinic she recently visited for pain in her right arm. The patient is married and lives with her husband and two grown children. According to the Uniform Health Care Decisions Act (UHCDA), who is the logical person to request and sign an authorization to access the woman's health records from the clinic?

    a. Adult child making request

    b. Oldest adult child

    c. Patient

    d. Spouse

393. Minors are basically deemed legally incompetent to access, use, or disclose their health information. What resource should be consulted in terms of who may authorize access, use, or disclose the health records of minors?

    a. HIPAA, because there are strict HIPAA rules regarding minors

    b. Hospital attorney since they know the rules of the hospital

    c. State law since HIPAA defers to state laws on matters related to minors

    d. State rules of evidence related to minors

394. The baby of a mother who is 15 years old was recently discharged from the hospital. The mother is seeking access to the baby's health record. Who must sign the authorization for release of the baby's health record?

    a. Both mother and father of the baby

    b. Maternal grandfather of the baby

    c. Maternal grandmother of the baby

    d. Mother of the baby

395. An employer has contacted the health information management department and requested health information on one of his employees. Of the options listed here, what is the best course of action?

    a. Provide the information requested.

    b. Refer the request to the attending physician.

    c. Request the employee's written authorization for release of information.

    d. Request the employer's written authorization for release of the employee's information.

396. The Latin phrase meaning "let the master answer" that puts responsibility for negligent actions of employees on the employer is called:

    a. *Res ipsalocquitor*

    b. *Res judicata*

    c. *Respondeat superior*

    d. *Restitutio in integrum*

397. Employees in the Hospital Business Office may have legitimate access to patient health information without patient authorization based on what HIPAA standard or principle?

    a. Minimum necessary

    b. Compound authorization

    c. Accounting of disclosures

    d. Preemption

398. Dr. Williams is on the medical staff of Sutter Hospital and he has asked to see the health record of his wife who was recently hospitalized. Dr. Jones was the patient's physician. Of the options listed here, which is the best course of action?

   a. Refer Dr. Williams to Dr. Jones and release the record if Dr. Jones agrees.

   b. Inform Dr. Williams that he cannot access his wife's health information unless she authorizes access through a written release of information.

   c. Request that Dr. Williams ask the hospital administrator for approval to access his wife's record.

   d. Inform Dr. Williams that he may review his wife's health record in the presence of the privacy officer.

399. In the situation of behavioral healthcare information, a healthcare provider may disclose health information on a patient without the patient's authorization in which of the following?

   a. Court order, duty to warn, and involuntary commitment proceedings

   b. Duty to warn, release of psychotherapy notes, and court order

   c. Involuntary commitment proceedings, court order, and substance abuse treatment records

   d. Release of psychotherapy notes, substance abuse treatment records, and duty to warn

400. What Act served to make electronic transactions as enforceable as paper transactions?

   a. Patient Self-Determination Act

   b. Uniform Electronic Transactions Act

   c. Health Care Quality Improvement Act

   d. Best Evidence Rule

401. Exceptions to the consent requirement include:

   a. Medical emergencies

   b. Provider discretion

   c. Implied consent

   d. Informed consent

402. When a patient revokes authorization for release of information *after* a healthcare facility has already released the information, the facility in this case:

   a. May be prosecuted for invasion of privacy

   b. Has become subject to civil action

   c. Has violated the security regulations of HIPAA

   d. Is protected by the Privacy Act

403. Generally, policies addressing the confidentiality of quality improvement (QI) committee data (minutes, actions, and so forth) state that this kind of data is:

   a. Protected from disclosure

   b. Subject to release with patient authorization

   c. Generally available to interested parties

   d. May not be reviewed or released to external reviewers such as the Joint Commission

404. Which one of the following has access to personally identifiable data without authorization or subpoena?

    a. Law enforcement in a criminal case

    b. The patient's attorney

    c. Public health departments for disease reporting purposes

    d. Workers' compensation for disability claim settlement

405. Under the HIPAA Privacy Rule, a hospital may disclose health information without authorization or subpoena in the following case:

    a. The patient has been involved in a crime that may result in death.

    b. The patient has celebrity status and requires protection.

    c. The father of a 22-year-old is requesting the records.

    d. An attorney requests records.

406. Under the HIPAA Privacy Rule, individuals have a right to do one of the following:

    a. Prohibit release of patient information for treatment reasons

    b. Refuse to pay reasonable copying costs

    c. Refuse release of reportable disease information

    d. Maintain all control over disclosure of information

407. Which one of the following facility types is required to release information under the Freedom of Information Act?

    a. Proprietary

    b. Military

    c. Private

    d. State

408. A hospital releases information to an insurance company with proper authorization by the patient. The insurance company forwards the information to a medical data clearinghouse. This process is referred to as:

    a. Admissibility

    b. Civil release

    c. Privileging process

    d. Redisclosure

409. A federal confidentiality statute specifically addresses confidentiality of health information about _____ patients.

    a. Developmentally disabled

    b. Elderly

    c. Drug and alcohol recovery

    d. Cancer

410. The confidentiality of incident reports is generally protected in cases where the report is filed in:

    a. The nursing notes

    b. The patient's health record

    c. The physician progress notes

    d. The hospital risk manager's office

411. Which of the following statements about the "legal health record" or the "designated record set" is incorrect?

    a. The designated record set is defined by HIPAA legislation.

    b. The legal health record is defined by the facility.

    c. The legal health record may not include all the information in the designated record set.

    d. The designated record set is determined by the medical staff.

412. The "Administrative Simplification" portion of Title II of HIPAA addresses one of the following:

    a. Creating standardized forms for release of information throughout the industry

    b. Computer memory requirements for health plans maintaining patient health information

    c. Security regulations for personal health records

    d. Uniform standards for transactions and code sets

413. An original goal of HIPAA Administrative Simplification was to standardize:

    a. Privacy notices given to patients

    b. The electronic transmission of health data

    c. Disclosure of information for treatment purposes

    d. The definition of PHI

414. Which of the following is an element that makes information "PHI" under the HIPAA Privacy Rule?

    a. Identifies an attending physician

    b. Specifies the insurance provider for the patient

    c. Contained within a personnel file

    d. Relates to one's health condition

415. Lane Hospital has a contract with Ready-Clean, a local company, to come into the hospital to pick up all the facility's linens for off-site laundering. Ready-Clean is:

    a. A business associate because Lane Hospital has a contract with it

    b. Not a business associate because it is a local company

    c. A business associate because its employees may see PHI

    d. Not a business associate because it does not use or disclose individually identifiable health information

416. Which of the following statements does the Privacy Rule require the Notice of Privacy Practices to contain?

    a. A description (including at least one example) of the types of uses and disclosures the physician is permitted to make for marketing purposes.

    b. A description of each of the other purposes for which the covered entity is permitted or required to use or disclose PHI without the individual's written consent or authorization.

    c. A statement that other uses and disclosures will be made without the individual's written authorization and that the individual may not revoke such authorization.

    d. A statement that all disclosures will be prohibited from future redisclosures.

417. Which of the following is a "public interest and benefit" exception to the authorization requirement?

    a. Payment

    b. PHI regarding victims of domestic violence

    c. Information requested by a patient's attorney

    d. Treatment

418. Central City Clinic has requested that Ghent Hospital send its hospital records from Susan Hall's most recent admission to the clinic for her follow-up appointment. Which of the following statements is true?

    a. The Privacy Rule requires that Susan Hall complete a written authorization.

    b. The hospital may send only discharge summary, history and physical, and operative report.

    c. The Privacy Rule's minimum necessary requirement does not apply.

    d. This "public interest and benefit" disclosure does not require the patient's authorization.

419. Under the Privacy Rule, the following must be included in a patient accounting of disclosures:

    a. State-mandated report of a sexually transmitted disease

    b. Disclosure pursuant to a patient's signed authorization

    c. Disclosure pursuant to meet national security or intelligence requirements

    d. Disclosure for payment purposes

420. Debbie, an HIM professional, was recently hired as the privacy officer at a large physician practice. She observes the following practices. Which is a violation of the HIPAA Privacy Rule?

    a. Dr. Graham recommends a medication to a patient with asthma.

    b. Dr. Herman gives a patient a pen with the name of a pharmaceutical company on it.

    c. Dr. Martin recommends acupuncture to a patient.

    d. Dr. Lawson gives names of asthma patients to a pharmaceutical company.

421. Per the Privacy Rule, which of the following requires authorization for research purposes?

    a. Use of Mary's information about her myocardial infarction, deidentified

    b. Use of Mary's information about her asthma, in a limited data set

    c. Use of Mary's individually identifiable information related to her asthma treatments

    d. Use of medical information about Jim, Mary's deceased husband

422. The HIPAA Privacy Rule permits charging patients for labor and supply costs associated with copying health records. Mercy Hospital is located in a state where state law allows charging patients a $100 search fee associated with locating records that have been requested. Which of the following statements is true when applied to this scenario?

    a. State law will not be preempted in this situation

    b. The Privacy Rule will preempt state law in this situation

    c. The Privacy Rule never preempts existing state law

    d. The Privacy Rule always preempts existing state law

423. Protected health information (PHI) that is maintained or transmitted in electronic form is called:

    a. aPHI

    b. Authenticated PHI

    c. Encrypted PHI

    d. ePHI

424. What is the most common method for implementing entity authentication?

    a. Personal identification number

    b. Biometric identification systems

    c. Token systems

    d. Password systems

425. An organization that is governed by the HIPAA regulations is called a(n):

    a. Authorized entity

    b. Covered entity

    c. Privacy entity

    d. Regulated entity

426. Which of the following is considered a two-factor authentication system?

    a. User ID with a password

    b. User ID with voice scan

    c. Password and swipe card

    d. Password and PIN

427. Which of the following statements about HIPAA training is false?

    a. Privacy and security training should be separated

    b. Different levels of training will be needed depending on an employee's position in the organization

    c. All employees in a healthcare organization need HIPAA training

    d. Training is required under the HIPAA Security Rule

428. Ted and Mary are the adoptive parents of Susan, a minor. What is the best way for them to obtain a copy of Susan's operative report?

    a. Wait until Susan is 18.

    b. Present an authorization signed by the court who granted the adoption.

    c. Present an authorization signed by Susan's natural (birth) parents.

    d. Present an authorization that at least one of them (Ted or Mary) has signed.

429. Many states have mandatory reporting requirements for suspected abuse or mistreatment of the following categories of individuals:

    a. Children, competent adults, and nursing home residents

    b. Competent adults, residents of mental health facilities, and nursing home residents

    c. Nursing home residents, the elderly, and residents of state mental health facilities

    d. Residents of state mental health facilities, the elderly, and competent adults

430. A subpoena *duces tecum* compels the recipient to:

    a. Serve on a jury

    b. Answer a complaint

    c. Testify at trial

    d. Bring records to a legal proceeding

431. The health record of Kathy Smith, the plaintiff, has been subpoenaed for a deposition. The plaintiff's attorney wants to use the records as evidence to prove his client's case. In this situation, although the record constitutes hearsay, it may be used as evidence based on the:

    a. Admissibility exception

    b. Discovery exception

    c. Direct evidence exception

    d. Business record exception

432. E-Discovery rules are amendments to the _____ and were created in response to the tremendous volume of evidence, maintained in electronic format, that is pertinent to lawsuits.

    a. Federal Rules of Evidence

    b. State Rules of Evidence

    c. Federal Rules of Civil Procedure

    d. State Rules of Civil Procedure

433. When a competent adult refuses treatment, a court may be required to balance the individual's privacy interests against the:

    a. Patient's level of pain

    b. Physician's right to keep the patient alive

    c. Government's interests in protecting human life

    d. Provider's liability concerns

434. A valid subpoena *duces tecum* seeking health records does not have to:

    a. Be signed by the plaintiff and defendant

    b. Include the date, time, and place of the requested appearance

    c. Include the case docket number

    d. Be accompanied by authorization from the patient whose records are sought

Domain VI *Legal and Regulatory Standards*

435. Which landmark legal case established the responsibility of the hospital for the quality of care given by its physicians?

    a. *Roe v. Wade*

    b. *Darling v. Charleston Community Memorial Hospital*

    c. *Brown v. Board of Education*

    d. *Marbury v. Madison*

436. What type of standard establishes clear descriptions of the data elements to be collected?

    a. Vocabulary standard

    b. Transaction and messaging standard

    c. Structure and content standard

    d. Security standard

437. Which of the following terms is used in reference to a written document that describes the patient's healthcare preferences in the event he or she becomes unable to communicate directly in the future?

    a. Interval note

    b. Rights statement

    c. Consent to treatment

    d. Advance directive

438. ASTM Standard E1384 provides guidance to healthcare organizations in developing:

    a. Data security

    b. Medical vocabulary

    c. Transaction standards

    d. Content and structure of health records

439. Laboratory data are successfully transmitted back and forth from Community Hospital to three local physician clinics. This successful transmission is dependent on which of the following standards?

    a. X12N

    b. LOINC

    c. RxNorm

    d. DICOM

440. Which of the following is an organization that develops standards related to healthcare delivery?

a. National Health Information Network

b. National Committee on Vital and Health Statistics

c. Health Level Seven

d. EHR Collaborative

441. In long-term care, the resident's care plan is based on data collected in the:

a. UHDDS

b. OASIS

c. MDS

d. HEDIS

442. Core immunization data elements to be included in an immunization registry were developed by the:

a. National Center for Health Statistics

b. American Health Information Management Association

c. Centers for Disease Control and Prevention

d. National Immunization Network

443. A radiology department is planning to develop a remote clinic and plans to transmit images for diagnostic purposes. The most important standards to implement in order to transmit images is:

a. X12N

b. LOINC

c. IEEE 1073

d. DICOM

444. What is it called when accrediting bodies such as the Joint Commission or AOA can survey facilities for compliance with the Medicare Conditions of Participation for Hospitals instead of the government?

a. Deemed status

b. Judicial decision

c. Subpoena

d. Credentialing

445. The name of the government agency that has led the development of basic data sets for health records and computer databases is the:

a. Centers for Medicare and Medicaid Services

b. Johns Hopkins University

c. American National Standards Institute

d. National Committee on Vital and Health Statistics

446. The four major issues that have an impact on the record retention policy of a healthcare facility are patient care, research, space, and:

a. Microfilm costs

b. Readmission rates

c. Destruction policy

d. Legal and statutory requirements

447. Accreditation standards and the Medicare Conditions of Participation require that the patient's _____ be documented by the attending physician in the patient's health record no more than 30 days after discharge.

a. Principal diagnosis

b. Principal procedure

c. Comorbidities

d. Complications

448. What term is used in reference to the systematic review of sample health records to determine whether documentation standards are being met?

a. Qualitative analysis

b. Legal record review

c. Quantitative analysis

d. Ongoing record review

449. According to the Joint Commission, the unanticipated death of a full-term infant should be reported as a(n):

a. Sentinel event

b. Violation of clinical practice guideline

c. Unfortunate accident

d. Medical accident

450. The _____ notifies physicians that Medicare payment to the facility is partly based on the patient's principal and secondary diagnoses, as well as the major procedures performed, and that falsification of records can lead to fines, imprisonment, or civil penalty under federal laws.

a. Medicare reimbursement rule

b. Physician acknowledgment statement

c. Provider agreement

d. Diagnosis and procedure validation statement

451. What is the first consideration in determining how long records must be retained?

a. The amount of space allocated for record filing

b. The number of records

c. The most stringent law or regulation in the state

d. The cost of filing space

452. Mary Smith delivers a stillborn infant at Medical Center Hospital. The appropriate method of documenting information about the infant is to:

    a. Create a health record for the infant

    b. File all infant information in the mother's record

    c. Retain the infant's information in a separate administrative file

    d. Not retain information about the infant in hospital records

453. Community Memorial Hospital is developing a new trauma center. The administrative team asks the director of HIM to ensure that hospital policies are in compliance with all regulations regarding acceptance and transfer of emergency patients. The legislation that the HIM director should review is the:

    a. Prospective Payment Act

    b. Health Insurance Portability and Accountability Act

    c. Emergency Medical Treatment and Active Labor Act

    d. Tax Equity and Fiscal Responsibility Act

454. A burn victim is brought to Community Memorial's new trauma center. There is no specialized burn care offered at Community Memorial, so the patient is stabilized and transferred 200 miles to a burn center with available beds. This situation is called a(n):

    a. Appropriate transfer

    b. Inappropriate transfer

    c. Dumping

    d. Palliative service

455. The Joint Commission requirement regarding delinquent records is that the number of delinquent records in a facility cannot exceed:

    a. 50 per week

    b. 2,000 per year

    c. 50% of the average number of discharges

    d. 25% of yearly admissions

456. The Joint Commission's position on autoauthentication of dictated and transcribed reports is which of the following?

    a. Fully supports

    b. Supports only for surgical dictation

    c. Supports only for discharge summaries

    d. Does not support

457. Dr. Smith dies while in solo medical practice. The best way to handle his patients' health records is to:

    a. Transfer each record to each patient's new attending physician

    b. Send all records to the local hospital for filing in its HIM department

    c. Destroy all records to avoid compromising confidential data

    d. Send all records to the state medical association for filing

458. If an HIM director wanted to access the rules and regulations regarding implementation of a federal law, where would he or she look?

a. *Congressional Register*

b. *Federal Register*

c. *Journal of American Health Information Management Association*

d. *Journal of American Medical Informatics Association*

459. How often annually are healthcare facilities required to practice their emergency preparedness plan?

a. Once

b. Twice

c. Three times

d. Never

460. This private, not-for-profit organization is committed to developing and maintaining practical, customer-focused standards to help organizations measure and improve the quality, value, and outcomes of behavioral health and medical rehabilitation programs.

a. Commission on Accreditation of Rehabilitation Facilities

b. American Osteopathic Association

c. National Committee for Quality Assurance

d. Joint Commission on Accreditation of Healthcare Organizations

PRACTICE EXAM 1

Domain I *Health Data Management*

1. Mildred Smith was admitted to a nursing facility with the following information: "Patient is being admitted for Organic Brain Syndrome." Underneath the diagnosis her medical information was listed along with her rehabilitation potential. This information is documented on the:

   a. Transfer or referral form

   b. Release of information form

   c. Patient's rights acknowledgment form

   d. Admitting physical evaluation form

2. A 65-year-old white male was admitted to the hospital on 1/15 complaining of abdominal pain. The Attending Physician requested an upper GI series and laboratory evaluation of CBC and UA. The x-ray revealed possible cholelithiasis and the UA showed an increased white blood cell count. The patient was taken to surgery for an exploratory laparoscopy and a ruptured appendix was discovered. The chief complaint was:

   a. Ruptured appendix

   b. Exploratory laparoscopy

   c. Abdominal pain

   d. Cholelithiasis

3. What type of data display tool is used to display discrete categories?

   a. Bar graph

   b. Histogram

   c. Pie chart

   d. Line chart

4. Using the following custom revenue production report, which coding error may be demonstrated in the report?

Revenue Production Report—Small Multispecialty Group Month: January				
Code	Quantity	Fee	Projected Revenue	Actual Insurance Revenue
99201	0	$50	$0	$0.00
99202	3	$75	$225	$164.10
99203	4	$90	$360	$267.94
99204	0	$120	$0	$0.00
99205	0	$150	$0	$.00
99211	703	$28	$19,684	$14,988.32
99212	489	$47	$22,983	$18,092.65
99213	1853	$63	$116,739	$92,890.38
99214	41	$89	$3,649	$2,799.11
99215	7	$135	$945	$722.87
99241	3	$100	$300	$52.50
99242	9	$125	$1,125	$156.23
99243	27	$150	$4,050	$610.45
99244	10	$175	$1,750	$124.32
99245	1	$200	$200	$53.10

a. Clustering

b. Unbundling

c. Missed charges

d. Overcoding

5. A system of names or terms used for a particular discipline created to facilitate communication by eliminating ambiguity is called:

a. Data dictionary

b. Clinical classification

c. Nomenclature

d. Clinical vocabulary

6. All documentation entered in the medical record relating to the patient's diagnosis and treatment are considered this type of data:

a. Clinical

b. Identification

c. Secondary

d. Financial

7. Data that have been grouped into meaningful categories according to a classification system are referred to as _____ data.

    a. Research

    b. Reference

    c. Coded

    d. Demographic

8. Before Central Hospital is permitted to open and provide medical services in a particular state, the organization must first go through which of the following processes?

    a. Accreditation

    b. Licensure

    c. Qualification

    d. Certification

9. What is the principal function of health records?

    a. Provide information for performance improvement activities

    b. Support billing and reimbursement processes

    c. Serve as the repository of clinical documentation relevant to the care of individual patients

    d. Determine appropriate resource allocation

10. What type of data is exemplified by the insured party's member identification number?

    a. Demographic data

    b. Clinical data

    c. Certification data

    d. Financial data

11. Which part of the problem-oriented medical record is used by many facilities who have not adopted the whole problem-oriented format?

    a. The problem list as an index

    b. The initial plan

    c. The SOAP form of progress notes

    d. The database

12. You are the coding supervisor and you are doing an audit of outpatient coding. Robert Thompson was seen in the outpatient department with a chronic cough and the record states, "rule out lung cancer." What should have been coded as the patient's diagnosis?

    a. Chronic cough

    b. Observation and evaluation without need for further medical care

    c. Diagnosis of unknown etiology

    d. Lung cancer

13. What type of patient information, when used in the aggregate, allows hospitals to draw comparisons across multiple health record sources?

    a. Administrative information

    b. Progress notes

    c. Demographic information

    d. Uniform data sets

14. Which of the following is a method of grouping patients according to a predefined set of characteristics?

    a. Case-mix analysis

    b. Case management

    c. Clinical practice guidelines

    d. Core measures

15. The _____ is/are used to gather information about specific health status factors and include(s) information about specific risk factors in the resident's care.

    a. Resident Assessment Protocols (RAP)

    b. Resident Assessment Instrument (RAI)

    c. Utilization Guidelines

    d. Minimum Data Set (MDS)

16. In the long-term care setting, these are problem-oriented frameworks for additional assessment based on problem identification items (triggered conditions).

    a. Resident Assessment Protocols (RAP)

    b. Resident Assessment Instrument (RAI)

    c. Utilization Guidelines (UG)

    d. Minimum Data Sets (MDS)

17. For Medicare patients, how often must the home health agency's assessment and care plan be updated?

    a. Every 60 days

    b. As often as the severity of the patient's condition requires

    c. At least every 60 days or as often as the severity of the patient's condition requires

    d. Every 30 days

18. A patient is admitted to an acute care hospital for acute intoxication and alcohol withdrawal syndrome due to chronic alcoholism.

291.8	Other specified alcohol-induced mental disorders
291.81	Other specified alcohol-induced mental disorders, alcohol withdrawal
303.00	Acute alcoholic intoxication, unspecified
305.00	Alcohol abuse, unspecified

a. 291.8, 303.00

b. 303.00

c. 305.00

d. 291.81, 303.00

19. A 45-year-old woman is admitted for blood loss anemia due to dysfunctional uterine bleeding.

218.9	Leiomyoma of uterus, unspecified
280.0	Iron deficiency anemias, secondary to blood loss (chronic)
285.1	Acute posthemorrhagic anemia
626.8	Disorders of menstruation and other abnormal bleeding from female genital tract, other

a. 280.0, 626.8

b. 285.1, 626.8

c. 626.8, 280.0

d. 280.0, 218.9

20. Patient is admitted with senile cataract; diabetes mellitus, and extracapsular cataract extraction with simultaneous insertion of intraocular lens.

250.00	Diabetes mellitus without mention of complication, type II or unspecified type, not stated as uncontrolled
250.50	Diabetes with ophthalmic manifestations, type II or unspecified type, not stated as uncontrolled
366.10	Senile cataract, unspecified
366.12	Incipient cataract
13.59	Other extracapsular extraction of lens
13.71	Insertion of intraocular lens prosthesis at time of cataract extraction, one-stage

a. 366.10, 250.50, 13.59, 13.71

b. 250.00, 366.10

c. 250.00, 366.12

d. 366.10, 250.00, 13.59, 13.71

21. A patient is admitted with acute exacerbation of COPD, chronic renal failure, and hypertension.

401.9	Essential hypertension, unspecified
403.10	Hypertensive chronic kidney disease, benign, with chronic kidney disease stage I through Stage IV, or unspecified
403.90	Hypertensive chronic kidney disease, unspecified, with chronic kidney disease stage I through stage IV, or unspecified
491.21	Obstructive chronic bronchitis, with (acute) exacerbation
492.8	Emphysema, other
496	Chronic airway obstruction, not elsewhere classified
585.9	Chronic kidney disease, unspecified

   a. 492.8, 496, 403.10, 585.9

   b. 492.8, 585.9, 401.9

   c. 496, 585.9, 401.9

   d. 491.21, 403.90, 585.9

22. Patient arrived via ambulance to the emergency department following a motor vehicle accident. Patient sustained a fracture of the ankle; 3.0 cm superficial laceration of the left arm; 5.0 laceration of the scalp with exposure of the fascia; and a concussion. Patient received the following procedures: x-ray of the ankle which showed a bimalleolar ankle fracture that required closed manipulative reduction and simple suturing of the arm laceration and layer closure of the scalp. Provide CPT codes for the procedures done in the emergency department for the facility bill.

12002	Simple repair of superficial wounds of scalp, neck, axillae, external genitalia, trunk and/or extremities (including hands and feet); 2.6 cm to 7.5 cm
12004	Simple repair of superficial wounds of scalp, neck, axillae, external genitalia, trunk and/or extremities (including hands and feet); 7.6 cm to 12.5 cm
12032	Repair, intermediate, wounds of scalp, axillae, trunk and/or extremities (excluding hands and feet); 2.6 cm to 7.5 cm
27810	Closed treatment of bimalleolar ankle fracture (eg, lateral and medial malleoli, or lateral and posterior malleoli, or medial and posterior malleoli); with manipulation
27818	Closed treatment of trimalleolar ankle fracture; with manipulation

   a. 27810, 12032

   b. 27818, 12004, 12032

   c. 27810, 12032, 12002

   d. 27810, 12004

23. The patient was admitted to the outpatient department and had a bronchoscopy with bronchial brushings performed.

	31622	Bronchoscopy, rigid or flexible, including fluoroscopic guidance, when performed, diagnostic, with cell washing when performed (separate procedure)
	31623	Bronchoscopy, rigid or flexible, including fluoroscopic guidance, when performed; with brushing or protected brushings
	31625	Bronchoscopy, rigid or flexible, including fluoroscopic guidance, when performed; with bronchial or endobronchial biopsy(s), single or multiple sites
	31640	Bronchoscopy, rigid or flexible, including fluoroscopic guidance, when performed; with excision of tumor

    a. 31622, 31640

    b. 31622, 31623

    c. 31623

    d. 31625

24. Identify the two-digit modifier that may be reported to indicate a physician performed the postoperative management of a patient, but another physician performed the surgical procedure.

    a. –22, Increased Procedural Services

    b. –54, Surgical Care Only

    c. –32, Mandated Service

    d. –55, Postoperative Management Only

25. What is the correct CPT code assignment for: destruction of internal hemorrhoids with use of infrared coagulation?

    a. 46255, Hemorrhoidectomy, internal and external, single column/group

    b. 46930, Destruction of internal hemorrhoid(s) by thermal energy (e.g., infrared coagulation, cautery, radiofrequency)

    c. 46260, Hemorrhoidectomy, internal and external, two or more columns/groups

    d. 46945, Hemorrhoidectomy, internal, by ligation other than rubber band; single hemorrhoid column/group

26. In data quality management, the process by which data elements are accumulated is:

    a. Warehousing

    b. Collection

    c. Application

    d. Analysis

27. The primary responsibility of a coder is to:

    a. Ensure timely processing of coded data

    b. Ensure quality of coded data

    c. Avoid claims rejections by third-party payers

    d. Ensure maximum reimbursement for the facility

28. A physician performed a total abdominal hysterectomy with bilateral salpingo-oophorectomy on his patient at Community Hospital. His office billed the following:

58150	Total abdominal hysterectomy with or without salpingo-oophorectomy
58720	Bilateral salpingo-oophorectomy

Why was this claim rejected?

a. Billed hysterectomy with wrong CPT code

b. Not a covered procedure

c. Unbundled procedures

d. Covered procedure but insurance company requires additional information

29. What part of the Medicare program was created under the Medicare Modernization Act of 2003 (MMA)?

a. Part A

b. Part B

c. Part C

d. Part D

30. A patient saw a neurosurgeon for treatment of a nerve that was severed in an industrial accident. The patient worked for Basic Manufacturing Company where the industrial accident occurred. Basic Manufacturing carried workers' compensation insurance. The workers' compensation insurance paid the fees of the neurosurgeon. Which entity is the "third party"?

a. Patient

b. Neurosurgeon

c. Basic Manufacturing Company

d. Workers' compensation insurance

31. The financial manager of the physician group practice explained that the healthcare insurance company would be reimbursing the practice for its treatment of the exacerbation of congestive heart failure that Mrs. Zale experienced. The exacerbation, treatment, and resolution covered approximately five weeks. The payment covered all the services that Mrs. Zale incurred during the period. What method of reimbursement was the physician group practice receiving?

a. Traditional

b. Episode-of-care

c. Per diem

d. Fee-for-service

32. The health plan reimburses Dr. Tan $15 per patient per month. In January, Dr. Tan saw 300 patients so he received $4,500 from the health plan. What method is the health plan using to reimburse Dr. Tan?

a. Traditional retrospective

b. Capitated rate

c. Relative value

d. Discounted fee schedule

33. New employee Jan Smith had worked for a manufacturing firm. While working for the manufacturing firm, she was covered under its group healthcare insurance for eight months. Jan terminated her employment with the manufacturing firm on a Friday and began a new position with a computer vendor the following Monday. The computer vendor also offers its employees a group healthcare plan. What is the maximum waiting period Jan should expect for her pre-existing condition?

> Preexisting conditions will be covered without a waiting period if:
> - An employee joins a new healthcare insurance group plan *and*
> - The employee had been insured for the previous 12 months under a group plan without a lapse in coverage exceeding 63 days.
>
> Preexisting conditions will be covered with a reduced waiting period if:
> - An employee joins a new healthcare insurance group plan *and*
> - The employee had previous creditable coverage without a lapse in coverage exceeding 63 days.
>
> The reduction equals the duration of the creditable coverage.

    a. 63 days

    b. 4 months

    c. 12 months

    d. Cannot be predicted

34. Which is the correct formula for wage index adjusting a payment?

    a. (payment rate $\times$ nonlabor portion $\times$ WI) + (payment rate $\times$ labor portion)

    b. (payment rate $\times$ labor portion $\times$ WI) + (payment rate $\times$ nonlabor portion)

    c. (payment rate $\times$ WI)

    d. (payment rate $\times$ nonlabor portion $\times$ WI) + (payment rate $\times$ labor rate $\times$ COLA)

35. The following table is an example of an:

Patient/Service	Service Date(s)	(A) Total Charge	(B) Not Payable by Plan		Plan Paid Amount	
White, Jane						
Office Visit	02/17/201X	$56.00	$10.00	CP*	$46.00	100%
X-Ray	02/17/201X	$268.00	$250.00 $3.60	DD* CI*	$14.40	80%
Lab	02/17/201X	$20.00	$15.00	CP*	$5.00	100%
Total						

CI: Coinsurance; CP: Copayment; DD: Deductible

    a. Explanation of benefits

    b. Insurance coverage advanced notice service waiver

    c. Insurance claim form

    d. Encounter form

36. Phil White had coronary artery bypass graft surgery. Unfortunately, during the surgery, Phil suffered a severe stroke. Phil's recovery included several settings in the continuum of care–acute-care hospital, physician office, rehabilitation center, and home health agency. This initial service and subsequent recovery lasted 10 months. As a member of an MCO in an integrated delivery system, how should Phil expect that his healthcare billing will be handled?

    a. Bills for each service from each physician, each facility, and each other healthcare provider from every encounter

    b. Bills for each service from each physician, each facility, and each other healthcare provider at the end of the 10-month period

    c. Consolidated billing for each encounter that includes the bills from all the physicians, facilities, and other healthcare providers involved in the encounter

    d. One fixed amount for the entire episode that is divided among all the physicians, facilities, and other healthcare providers

Domain II *Health Statistics and Research Support*

37. In which of the following phases of systems selection and implementation would the process of running a mock query to assess the functionality of a database be performed?

    a. Initial study

    b. Design

    c. Testing

    d. Operation

38. A health information professional is preparing statistical information about the third-party payers that reimburse care in the facility. She finds the following information: Medicare reimburses 46 percent; Medicaid reimburses 13 percent; Blue Cross reimburses 21 percent; workers' compensation reimburses 1 percent; commercial plans reimburse 15 percent; and other payers or self-payers reimburse 4 percent. What is the best graphic tool to use to display this data?

    a. Histogram

    b. Pie chart

    c. Line graph

    d. Table

39. During an influenza outbreak, a nursing home reports 25 new cases of influenza in a given month. These 25 cases represent 30 percent of the nursing home's population. This rate represents the:

    a. Prevalence

    b. Incidence

    c. Frequency

    d. Distribution

40. Which of the following conditions would be the most likely to fall into the category of notifiable diseases as defined by the National Notifiable Diseases Surveillance System?

    a. Diabetes mellitus

    b. Coronary artery disease

    c. Fracture of major bones

    d. HIV infection

41. What is the formatting problem in the following table?

Medical Center Hospital Admission Types		
Elective	2,843	62.4
Emergency admission	942	37.6
Total	3,785	100.0

    a. Variable names are missing.

    b. The title of the table is missing.

    c. The column headings are missing.

    d. The column totals are inaccurate.

42. The following data have been collected by the hospital quality council. What conclusions can be made from the data on the hospital's quality of care between the first and second quarters?

Measure	1st Qtr	2nd Qtr
Medication errors	3.2%	10.4%
Patient falls	4.2%	8.6%
Hospital-acquired infections	1.8%	4.9%
Transfusion reactions	1.4%	2.5%

    a. Quality of care improved between the first and second quarters

    b. Quality of care is about the same between the first and second quarters

    c. Quality of care is declining between the first and second quarters

    d. Quality of care should not be judged by these types of measures

43. Using the admission criteria provided, determine if the following patient meets severity of illness and intensity of service criteria for admission.

Severity of Illness	Intensity of Service
Persistent fever	Inpatient-approved surgery/procedure within 24 hours of admission
Active bleeding	Intravenous medications and/or fluid replacement
Wound dehiscence	Vital signs every 2 hours or more often

Sue presents with vaginal bleeding. An ultrasound showed a missed abortion so she is being admitted to the outpatient surgery suite for a D&C.

a. The patient does not meet both severity of illness and intensity of service criteria.

b. The patient does meet both severity of illness and intensity of service criteria.

c. The patient meets intensity of service criteria but not severity of illness.

d. The patient meets severity of illness criteria but not intensity of service.

44. If a child was admitted to a hospital with a fever and within 24 hours developed measles, the measles would be classified as:

a. Healthcare-associated infection

b. Hospital sickness

c. Community-acquired infection

d. Community sickness

45. The surgery department is evaluating its postoperative infection rate of 6 percent. The chief of surgery asks the quality improvement coordinator to find the postoperation infection rates of 10 similar hospitals in the same geographic region to see how the rates compare. This process is called:

a. Universal precautions

b. Internal comparisons

c. Benchmarking

d. Critical pathway analysis

46. One of the roles of the health information professional in clinical quality management is:

a. Performing safety checks on new equipment

b. Training physicians on new surgical procedures

c. Making judgments about the quality of clinical care

d. Interpreting data in a meaningful way

47. In assessing the quality of care given to patients with diabetes mellitus, the CQI group collects data regarding blood sugar levels on admission and on discharge. This data is called a(n):

a. Indicator

b. Measurement

c. Assessment

d. Outcome

48. The Universal Protocol requires a "time-out" prior to the start of any surgical or invasive procedure to conduct a verification of:

    a. Patient and procedure

    b. Patient, procedure, and site

    c. Surgeon and site

    d. Surgeon, patient, and site

49. For the following excerpt from a patient satisfaction survey, determine if, in the development of this survey, the designer is adhering to good survey design principles.

    ```
    What is your zip code? _____
    Sex (circle one):       Male       Female
    What is your age?
       0–17 _____
      18–35 _____
      36–45 _____
      46–60 _____
    ```

    a. All survey design principles were applied in the development of this survey.

    b. The survey design principle of consistent format was applied in the development of this survey.

    c. The survey design principle of mutually exclusive categories was applied in the development of this survey.

    d. The survey design principles were not applied in the development of this survey.

50. Using the staff turnover information in this graph, determine what the next action the Quality Council at this hospital should take.

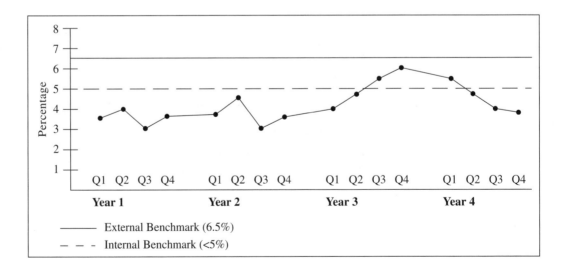

    a. Nothing, as the data is below the external benchmark.

    b. Coordinate a PI team to look into the cause for the high employee turnover rate in year 3.

    c. Coordinate a PI team to look into the cause for the drop in employee turnover rate in year 4.

    d. Nothing, as the data is above the internal benchmark.

51. Which of the following processes would investigate a medical error that resulted in the death of a patient?

    a. Security management

    b. Risk management

    c. Diagnostic review

    d. Accreditation

52. Community Memorial Hospital discharged nine patients on April 1st. The length of stay for each patient is shown in the following table. The average length of stay for these nine patients was:

Patient	Number of Days
A	1
B	5
C	3
D	3
E	8
F	8
G	8
H	9
I	9

    a. 5 days

    b. 6 days

    c. 8 days

    d. 9 days

53. In large research institutions, informed consent forms are generally monitored by the:

    a. Chief of staff

    b. CIO

    c. Institutional Review Board (IRB)

    d. Health information management professional

54. Rates for population-based statistics are reported per 1,000, 10,000, or 100,000 individuals. Rates for healthcare facility statistics are reported per _____ cases.

    a. 100

    b. 1,000

    c. 10,000

    d. 100,000

55. Which of the following would be an indicator of process problems in a health information department?

    a. 5% decline in the number of patients who indicate satisfaction with hospital care

    b. 10% increase in the average length of stay

    c. 15% reduction in bed turnover rate

    d. 18% error rate on abstracting data

56. What is the biggest problem with using mean length of stay as a facility statistic?

    a. It is not accurate.

    b. It is influenced by outlier values.

    c. It is mathematically incorrect.

    d. It is a dependent variable.

Domain III *Information Technology and Systems*

57. Which of the following best describes the intent of strategic information systems planning?

    a. Provide the potential for growth and expansion

    b. Ensure that all IS technology initiatives are integrated and aligned with the organization's overall strategy

    c. Assess community/market needs and resources

    d. Ensure ongoing accreditation

58. Which of the following are phases of the systems development life cycle (SDLC)?

    a. Design, analysis, and alignment

    b. Maintenance, implementation, and improvement

    c. Analysis, design, and implementation

    d. Analysis, alignment, and improvement

59. Which of the following activities is likely to occur in the analysis phase of the systems development life cycle?

    a. Examine current system and identify opportunities for improvement

    b. Send out RFPs to prospective vendors

    c. Negotiate contract with vendor

    d. Install necessary hardware and software

60. Assume you are the manager of a 10-physician group primary care practice. The physicians are interested in contracting with an application service provider to develop and manage patient records electronically. Which of the following statements is an indication that an ASP may be a good idea for this practice?

    a. The practice does not have the upfront capital or IT staff needed to purchase and implement a system from a health information systems vendor.

    b. The practice wants an electronic medical record system and wants to get into the IT management business as well.

    c. The practice would like to have the system up and running in a relatively short period of time (less than four months).

    d. The practice is not looking to purchase any additional hardware needed for an electronic medical record system.

61. Which one of the following statements most accurately describes the optimal relationship between strategic planning and strategic IS planning in a healthcare organization?

    a. There is no relationship. The two processes should occur separately and independent of one another; otherwise, the "waters can get murky."

    b. The strategic IS planning process should be done first. The organization's overall strategic directions should then emerge from the IS planning process.

    c. The two processes are clearly related. It is important for the CIO to be involved in both processes to ensure that IS priorities are congruent with the overall strategic plans of the organization.

    d. The two processes are clearly related. However, the CIO should not be involved in the overall strategic planning process. Having the CIO there might steer the discussion to technology and that should not occur at this stage in the process.

62. Among the following, who on the IT department staff would likely have as part of his/her position description "design, test, and evaluate LAN, Internet, and intranets"?

    a. Database administrator

    b. Network administrator

    c. Telecommunications specialist

    d. Systems analyst

63. At Medical Center Hospital, the master patient index system is not meeting facility needs. There are duplicate numbers and errors in patient identification information. The IS director replaces the system with a newer system from a different vendor. After several months, the new system is exhibiting many of the same problems as the old system, and the facility staff is frustrated and angry. What is the most likely cause of the problem?

    a. The new system has the same design flaws as the previous system.

    b. The old system was not properly disabled and has infected the new system.

    c. Underlying human and process problems were not identified and corrected prior to making a system change.

    d. Human error is the cause of all of the problems with both systems.

64. A health information exchange organization that has no access to personal health information is an example of this kind of architectural model:

    a. Consolidated

    b. Federated—consistent database

    c. Federated—inconsistent databases

    d. Switch

65. What is the data model that is most widely used to illustrate a relational database structure?

    a. Unified medical language ML

    b. Entity-relationship diagram

    c. Object model

    d. Relational model

66. Which of the following is an example of an M:M relationship?

    a. Patients to hospital admissions

    b. Patients to consulting physicians

    c. Patients to hospital medical records

    d. Primary care physicians to patients

67. This type of network uses a private tunnel through the Internet as a transport medium.

    a. Virtual privacy network

    b. Local area network

    c. Wide area network

    d. Intranet

68. Using the information in these partial attribute lists for the PATIENT, VISIT, and CLINIC columns in a relational database, the attribute PATIENT_MRN is listed in both the PATIENT Entity Attributes and the VISIT Entity Attributes, and CLINIC_ID is listed in both the VISIT Entity Attributes and the CLINIC Entity Attributes. What does the attribute PATIENT_MRN represent?

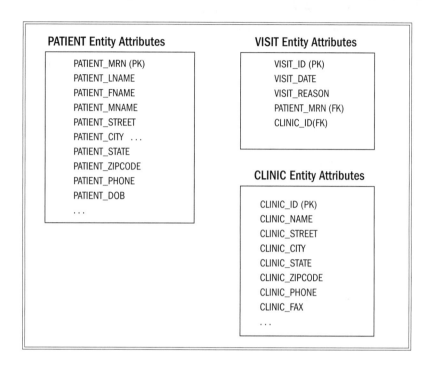

PATIENT Entity Attributes

PATIENT_MRN (PK)
PATIENT_LNAME
PATIENT_FNAME
PATIENT_MNAME
PATIENT_STREET
PATIENT_CITY . . .
PATIENT_STATE
PATIENT_ZIPCODE
PATIENT_PHONE
PATIENT_DOB
. . .

VISIT Entity Attributes

VISIT_ID (PK)
VISIT_DATE
VISIT_REASON
PATIENT_MRN (FK)
CLINIC_ID(FK)

CLINIC Entity Attributes

CLINIC_ID (PK)
CLINIC_NAME
CLINIC_STREET
CLINIC_CITY
CLINIC_STATE
CLINIC_ZIPCODE
CLINIC_PHONE
CLINIC_FAX
. . .

a. It is the foreign key in PATIENT and the primary key in VISIT.

b. It is the primary key in PATIENT and the foreign key in VISIT.

c. It is the primary key in both PATIENT and VISIT.

d. It is the foreign key in both PATIENT and VISIT.

69. Anywhere Hospital has mandated that the social security number will be displayed in the XXX-XX-XXXX format for their patients. This is an example of the use of a:

a. Wildcard

b. Mask

c. Truncation

d. Data definition

70. Which organization has created a standard for EHR system functions?

a. AHIMA

b. Federal government

c. HL7

d. IOM

71. In which form of database would complex data analysis most effectively take place?

    a. Clinical data repository

    b. Clinical data warehouse

    c. Database management system

    d. Electronic health record

72. Which of the following is a system in which the patient health record is kept in the same order on the nursing station and in the complete record?

    a. Standard

    b. Universal

    c. Source-oriented

    d. Patient-centered

73. Data that are collected on large populations of individuals and stored in databases are referred to as:

    a. Statistics

    b. Information

    c. Aggregate data

    d. Standards

74. Which national database includes data on all discharged patients regardless of payer?

    a. Healthcare Cost and Utilization Project

    b. Medicare Provider Analysis and Review file

    c. Unified Medical Language System

    d. Uniform Hospital Discharge Data Set

75. An encoder that takes a coder through a series of questions and choices is called a(n):

    a. Automated codebook

    b. Automated code assignment

    c. Logic-based encoder

    d. Decision support database

76. What does an audit trail check for?

    a. Unauthorized access to a system

    b. Loss of data

    c. Presence of a virus

    d. Successful completion of a backup

77. Healthcare organizations and practitioners throughout the country need a common terminology that is integrated into the electronic health record to:

    a. Read tests more accurately

    b. Exchange and use information reliably

    c. Prepare secondary records

    d. Track population mortality

78. An individual designated as an inpatient coder may have access to an electronic medical record in order to code the record. Under what access security mechanism is the coder allowed access to the system?

    a. Role-based

    b. User-based

    c. Context-based

    d. Situation-based

79. Which of the following statements about a firewall is false?

    a. It is a system or combination of systems that supports an access control policy between two networks.

    b. The most common place to find a firewall is between the healthcare organization's internal network and the Internet.

    c. Firewalls are effective for preventing all types of attacks on a healthcare system.

    d. A firewall can limit internal users from accessing various portions of the Internet.

80. An audit trail is a good tool for which one of the following?

    a. Holding an individual patient accountable for actions

    b. Reconstructing electronic events

    c. Defending the corporation against an IRS audit

    d. Stopping attacks from the intranet to the Internet

81. The data elements in a patient's automated laboratory result are examples of:

    a. Unstructured data

    b. Free-text data

    c. Financial data

    d. Structured data

82. Which of the following is an example of analog data?

    a. CT scan

    b. Photographic, chest x-ray film

    c. MRI exam

    d. EKG tracing

83. The technology that considers syntax, semantics, and context to accurately process and extract speech data is:

    a. Boolean word search

    b. Speech recognition technology

    c. Continuous speech input

    d. Natural language processing

84. The personal health record model that maintains provider control on content while allowing online access to the authorized patient is the:

   a. Shared data record model

   b. EHR extension model

   c. Provider-sponsored information management model

   d. Smart card model

85. The technology commonly utilized for automated claims processing (sending bills directly to third-party payers) is:

   a. Optical character recognition

   b. Bar coding

   c. Neural networks

   d. Electronic data interchange

86. Technology that electronically stores, manages, and distributes documents that are generated in a digital format and whose output data are report-formatted is called:

   a. Business process management (BPM) technology

   b. Automated forms processing technology

   c. Computer output laser disk (COLD) technology

   d. Digital signature management technology

87. University Medical Center contracts with the XYZ Corporation for a clinical information system. The hospital pays a fixed monthly fee. XYZ owns the hardware and hosts the application software using the Internet. The Medical Center accesses the system through onsite workstations. In this situation, XYZ Corporation is a(n):

   a. Application service provider

   b. Neural network

   c. Health information system database

   d. Clinician portal

88. Often considered the most important resource in a healthcare facility, this index is a database of patients within a facility or associated group of facilities.

   a. Facility-specific index

   b. Master patient index

   c. Disease index

   d. Disease and operation index

89. What type of authentication is created when a person signs his or her name on a pen pad and the signature is automatically converted and affixed to a computer document?

   a. Digital signature

   b. Electronic validation

   c. Electronic signature

   d. Electronic authorization key

90. An internal link that allows only the employees of a particular organization to navigate and communicate in a web-based environment is a(n):

    a. Internet

    b. Repository

    c. Intranet

    d. Access code

91. The application of information science to the management of healthcare data and information through computer technology is referred to as:

    a. Data definitions

    b. Data resource management

    c. Healthcare informatics

    d. Clinical information systems

92. What type of safeguard is more people-focused in nature?

    a. Technical

    b. Administrative

    c. Physical

    d. Addressable

Domain IV *Organization and Management*

93. External change agents have the advantage over internal agents of:

    a. Benchmarking the organization against other organizations

    b. Being less objective

    c. Understanding the history of the organization

    d. Being less expensive to employ

94. Bob Smith was admitted to Mercy Hospital on June 21. The physical was completed on June 23. According to Joint Commission standards, which statement applies to this situation?

    a. The record is not in compliance as the physical exam must be completed within 24 hours of admission.

    b. The record is not in compliance as the physical exam must be completed within 48 hours of admission.

    c. The record is in compliance as the physical exam must be completed within 48 hours.

    d. The record is in compliance as the physical exam was completed within 72 hours of admission.

95. Employees covered by the provisions of the Fair Labor Standards Act (FLSA) are called _____ employees.

    a. Waged

    b. Salaried

    c. Exempt

    d. Nonexempt

96. A work schedule that requires employees to be at their job between 10:00 a.m. and 2:00 p.m. but permits them to vary their schedule during the rest of the day to fit their needs is called:

    a. A compressed workweek

    b. Flextime

    c. Telecommuting

    d. Job sharing

97. Appreciative inquiry involves:

    a. Adjusting leadership style to the developmental stages of a team

    b. Finding organizational processes that already work and adapting them for use elsewhere

    c. Using interpersonal skills to discover reasons for resistance to change

    d. Using charisma to influence others

98. The "glass ceiling" refers to:

    a. The highest level of achievement to which a leader can aspire

    b. The limits of promotion that a member of the "in-group" can attain

    c. The implicit barriers that prevent certain groups from promotion in the organization

    d. Organizational effort to diversify the workforce

99. According to the records kept on filing unit performance over the past year, the filing unit has filed an average of 1,000 records per day. You have three FTE record filers in the department who are productive 88 percent of each workday (that is, 12 percent unproductive or 12 percent PFD). Based on this information, what is the average number of records filed per productive hour in the file unit as a whole?

    a. 42 charts/hour

    b. 48 charts/hour

    c. 110 charts/hour

    d. 143 charts/hour

100. The slightly higher wage paid to an employee who works a less desirable shift is called a:

    a. Shift rotation

    b. Performance incentive

    c. Shift differential

    d. Work distribution ladder

101. A summary of the responsibilities of a position, a list of duties, and a list of qualifications required to perform the job are all elements of a(n):

    a. Orientation plan

    b. Performance review

    c. Position description

    d. Schedule

102. How are employee performance standards used?

    a. To communicate performance expectations

    b. To assign daily work

    c. To describe the elements of a job

    d. To prepare a job advertisement

103. Which of the following statements is most accurate regarding communication errors?

    a. Incompetence is at the root of most communication errors.

    b. One error usually contributes to a chain of additional errors.

    c. Communication errors between managers and staff is nearly negligible.

    d. Message content is more important than how it is delivered.

104. The form of coaching in which an individual in the beginning stages of a career is matched as a protégé with a senior person is known as:

    a. Mentoring

    b. Cross-training

    c. Orientation

    d. Motivation

105. A set of activities designed to familiarize new employees with their jobs, the organization, and the work culture is called:

    a. Training

    b. Job analysis

    c. Job rotation

    d. Orientation

106. Which of the following payment arrangements is streamlined by the use of Chargemasters?

    a. Fee-for-service

    b. Per diem

    c. Prospective

    d. Retrospective

107. A risk of an organization being driven by charismatic leadership is that:

    a. They are more concerned with vision than productivity

    b. Motivation may decline with the loss of the leader

    c. The leader does not encourage sufficient commitment from workers

    d. There is low faith in the organizational vision

108. Synergy refers to:

   a. The combination of everyone's effort accomplishes more than each person acting alone

   b. The inevitable decline in performance as an organization ages

   c. One of the effects of groupthink

   d. What occurs when the management behavior does not fit the person to whom it is applied

109. The following performance standard, "Respond to release of information requests for continuing care in one working day 95 percent of the time," is an example of a:

   a. Quality standard

   b. Quantity standard

   c. Joint Commission standard

   d. Compliance standard

110. A coding service had 400 discharged records to code in March. The service coded 200 within 3 days, 100 within 5 days, 50 within 8 days, and 50 within 10 days. The average TAT for coding in March was:

   a. 3 days

   b. 5 days

   c. 6.5 days

   d. 9 days

111. What term is used to represent a difference between the budgeted amount and the actual amount of a line item that is expected to reverse itself during a subsequent period?

   a. Permanent variance

   b. Fixed cost

   c. Temporary variance

   d. Flexible cost

112. What basic accounting principle requires that helpful explanations accompany financial reports, when necessary?

   a. Disclosure

   b. Reliability

   c. Matching

   d. Consistency

113. Trinity Hospital has a fiscal year end of August 31. For this hospital, the second quarter ends:

   a. November 30

   b. February 28 or 29

   c. May 31

   d. August 31

114. Virtually every financial transaction consists of three fundamental steps. These steps include:

    a. Goods or services are provided, compensation is exchanged, and the balance sheet is adjusted

    b. A transaction is recorded, the balance sheet is adjusted, and a cost analysis is performed

    c. Compensation is exchanged, a cost analysis is performed, and a transaction is recorded

    d. A transaction is recorded, compensation is exchanged, and goods or services are provided

115. Dr. Blake's administrative assistant purchased office supplies at an office supplies store and charged the purchase to the doctor's account. The journal entry used to record this transaction is a debit to office supplies expense and a credit to:

    a. Purchases

    b. Cash

    c. Accounts payable

    d. Revenue

116. The following information was abstracted from Community Hospital's balance sheet.

Total assets	$25,000,000
Current assets	$4,000,000
Total liabilities	$10,000,000
Current liabilities	$5,000,000

A vendor selling a large-dollar amount of goods to this hospital on credit would:

    a. Not be concerned because total assets exceed total liabilities

    b. Not be concerned because the debt ratio is less than one half

    c. Be somewhat concerned because the current ratio is less than one

    d. Not analyze the balance sheet because the vendor would care more about the income statement

117. The HIM department records copy fees as revenue. Year-to-date, the budgeted fees are $25,000 and the actual fees received are $23,000. The director may be asked to explain a(n):

    a. Favorable variance of $2,000

    b. Unfavorable variance of $2,000

    c. Favorable variance of $23,000

    d. Unfavorable variance of $23,000

118. Community Hospital is purchasing a new ambulance. The ambulance will cost $100,000, which will be depreciated at $20,000 per year for five years. Related cash inflows from reimbursements are projected to be $80,000 annually. The hospital expects to replace the vehicle when it is fully depreciated. How much is the accounting rate of return on this investment?

    a. 20%

    b. 40%

    c. 60%

    d. 80%

119. In 1980, Community Hospital purchased a building for its clinic for $200,000. In 2002, the hospital sold the building for $850,000.

Accounting Rate of Return	
Investment	$100,000
Straight-Line Depreciation over 5 years	$20,000 per year
Cash In	$80,000 per year
ARR	60% [(80,000 − 20,000) / 100,000]

The return on this investment (ROI) is:

a. 24%

b. 76%

c. 325%

d. 425%

120. Community Hospital is evaluating the following three investments. Which one has the highest profitability index?

	Radiology Investment	Cardiology Investment	Pharmacy Investment
Present value of cash inflows	$2,000,000	$1,200,000	$40,000
Present value of cash outflows	$500,000	$300,000	$10,000

a. Radiology investment

b. Cardiology investment

c. Pharmacy investment

d. All three are equally profitable

Use the following information for questions 121 through 123:

> At the end of March, the HIM department has a YTD payroll budget of $100,000. The actual YTD amount paid is $95,000 because a coder resigned in February. For the past two months, the position has been filled through outsourcing. Therefore, the actual YTD amount for consulting services is $5,000, although no money was budgeted for consulting services. The reporting threshold for variances is 4%. The fiscal year-end is December.

121. What is the best description of the payroll variance for this year?

a. Favorable, permanent

b. Unfavorable, permanent

c. Favorable, temporary

d. Unfavorable, temporary

122. What is the best description of the consulting services variance?

   a. Favorable, permanent

   b. Unfavorable, permanent

   c. Favorable, temporary

   d. Unfavorable, temporary

123. Which one of the variances will the HIM director be required to explain?

   a. Only the consulting services variance

   b. Only the payroll variance

   c. Both the payroll and consulting services variances

   d. Neither because the two variances cancel each other out

124. Seaside Hospital is a small, private acute-care facility owned and operated by a recognized religious organization. Which of the following sources of accounting and reporting rules will apply to Seaside?

   a. FASB, SEC, IRS, PCAOB, CMS

   b. SEC, IRS, PCAOB

   c. FASB, IRS, SEC, CMS

   d. FASB, IRS, CMS

125. The time required to recoup the cost of an investment is called the:

   a. Accounting rate of return

   b. Budget cycle

   c. Payback period

   d. Depreciation

126. Dr. Phillips, Dr. Patel, and Dr. Blankley are all gynecologists. They work together under the name Community Women's Center. Dr. Phillips owns 50 percent of the business. Dr. Patel and Dr. Blankley each own 25 percent of the business. The profits from their business flow directly to their personal tax returns. The doctors would like to bring another practitioner into the business as an owner. Which of the following actions must take place in order to bring a new owner into the business?

   a. The existing owners must each sell some of their shares to the new owner.

   b. The existing owners must dissolve the existing partnership and make a new partnership agreement.

   c. The new practitioner must come in as an employee.

   d. The Board of Trustees must authorize a resolution to accept a new partner.

127. The idea that leaders are born, not made is most related to:

   a. Great Person theory

   b. LMX theory

   c. Contingency theory

   d. Path-Goal theory

128. A person who described a leader as being attractive, verbally fluent, creative, assertive, and a good team player would be using which theory?

    a. Path-Goal theory

    b. Theory X-Y

    c. Maturity theory

    d. Trait theory

129. The advantage of using internal change agents over external change agents is that the former can usually:

    a. Be accepted by employees as being more objective

    b. Provide a more detailed understanding of organizational history and issues

    c. More easily challenge organizational norms and culture

    d. Benchmark the organization against others

130. One of the differences between leaders and managers is that leaders more often:

    a. Have more turbulence in their early lives

    b. Are strongly dependent on others for their security

    c. Pay attention to present efficiency

    d. Use structured and analytical thinking

131. Which of the following is a characteristic of storytelling as a creative technique?

    a. Most people are uncomfortable with this approach.

    b. It is familiar and understandable.

    c. Stories are hard to develop and hard to remember.

    d. It rallies a group to take action.

132. Tichy describes three organizational components that must be managed in the change process. What are they?

    a. Technical, political, and social

    b. Technical, political, and cultural

    c. Political, social, and managerial

    d. Cultural, political, and human

133. Which of the following system components allows one to determine whether the results that were actually achieved are the results that were expected?

    a. Inputs

    b. Process

    c. Outputs

    d. Feedback

134. Which of the following is a true statement about business process reengineering?

    a. It is intended to make small incremental changes to improve a process.

    b. It seeks to reevaluate and redesign organizational processes to make dramatic performance improvements.

    c. It implies making few changes to achieve significant improvements in cost, quality, service, and speed.

    d. Its main focus is to reduce services.

135. Coders at Medical Center Hospital are expected to do a high volume of coding. Their department also includes a clerical support person who handles phone calls, pulls and files records to be coded, and maintains productivity logs. An abstract clerk enters coded data into the health information system. This is an example of _____ work division.

    a. Parallel

    b. Unit

    c. Serial

    d. Serial unit

136. What is change control used for in project management?

    a. Handing off deliverables from one team member to another

    b. Managing scope modifications

    c. Determining the project dependencies

    d. Documenting the project organizational chart

137. In the following figure, identify the component of the project plan labeled as B.

A				1/12	1/13	1/14	1/15	1/16	1/19	1/20
1.	🗎	1. Test ADT-Lab interface		C						
2.		1.1 Write test scenario	Dr. Smith							
					D					
3.	✓ B	1.2 Load test data	John					E		
4.		1.3 Execute lab order	Mary							

    a. Row numbers

    b. Task completed

    c. Task progress

    d. Dependency

138. A director of health information services in a hospital wants to implement a computer-based patient record system over the next two years. She gets support from the CIO, who champions the project with the administrative team. The CIO has become the project's:

    a. Stakeholder

    b. Sponsor

    c. Manager

    d. Budget director

139. An organization plans to implement an EHR project in which nurses will electronically document their observations and treatments. It is thought that hand-held personal digital assistants, rather than laptop computers or bedside terminals, will be used for this function. This type of prediction is called a(n):

    a. Parameter

    b. Assumption

    c. Scope

    d. Delimiter

140. Reviewing the following PERT chart, what is the critical path for this project?

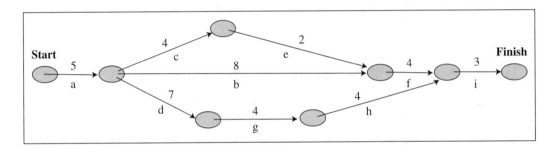

    a. a → c → d → f → i

    b. a → b → f → i

    c. a → d → g → h → i

    d. a → c → e → f → i

141. A small physician practice acquired EHR software. The vendor was contracted to conduct the software installation. One of the physicians installed the hardware the weekend prior to the vendor coming on-site. On the day the vendor arrived, a nurse was asked to sit with the vendor and explain the office's clinical processes. After the first week, a member of the IT department at the hospital was asked to assist the office because the portal to the hospital was not working correctly. At the end of the second week, the office manager was fired because two prescriptions faxed to the local pharmacy did not get received. What is the cause of the unsuccessful start-up of this implementation?

    a. Lack of priority

    b. Lack of sponsorship

    c. Lack of ownership

    d. Lack of project manager

142. A community hospital recently signed a contract for an EHR. The steering committee has now split up into respective domains, so that nurses are working on medication administration, physicians on order entry, HIM on document management, patient financial services on revenue cycle, etc. When the nurses were ready to implement medication administration, however, they found that they could only implement part of the process because the pharmacy had not yet completed its unit-dosing project. What is the cause of the unplanned interruption of implementation?

    a. Lack of priority

    b. Lack of sponsorship

    c. Lack of ownership

    d. Lack of project manager

143. The leader of the coding performance improvement team wants all team members to clearly understand the coding process. What tool could help accomplish this objective?

    a. Flowchart

    b. Force-field analysis

    c. Pareto chart

    d. Scatter diagram

144. Once all data has been posted to patient's account, the claim can be reviewed for accuracy and completeness. Many facilities have an internal auditing system that runs each claim through a set of edits. This internal auditing system is known as a:

    a. Chargemaster

    b. Superbill

    c. Scrubber

    d. Grouper

145. Contracting for staffing to handle a complete function within the HIM department, for example, the Cancer Registry function, would be consider what type of contracting arrangement?

    a. Full-service

    b. Part-time service

    c. Project based

    d. Temporary

146. Every year, a director of health information services sponsors a series of presentations about the confidentiality of patient information. All facility employees are required to attend a session. This method of educational delivery is called:

    a. Career development

    b. In-service education

    c. On-the-job training

    d. Orientation

Domain V *Privacy, Security, and Confidentiality*

147. When a patient collapses upon arrival at the entrance to an emergency department, what type of treatment authorization is in effect?

    a. Emergency consent

    b. Implied consent

    c. Informed consent

    d. Expressed consent

148. What should a hospital do when a state law requires more stringent privacy protection than the federal HIPAA privacy standard?

    a. Ignore the state law and follow the HIPAA standard

    b. Follow the state law and ignore the HIPAA standard

    c. Comply with both the state law and the HIPAA standard

    d. Ignore both the state law and the HIPAA standard and follow relevant accreditation standards

149. Which legal doctrine was established by the *Darling v. Charleston Community Hospital* case of 1965?

    a. Hospital–physician negligence

    b. Clinical negligence

    c. Physician–hospital negligence

    d. Corporate negligence

150. Which national database was created to collect information on the legal actions (both civil and criminal) taken against licensed healthcare providers?

    a. Healthcare Integrity and Protection Data Bank

    b. Medicare Protection Database

    c. National Practitioner Data Bank

    d. Healthcare Safety Database

151. Mary Smith has gone to her doctor to discuss her current medical condition. What is the legal term that best describes the type of communication that has occurred between Mary and her physician?

    a. Closed communication

    b. Open communication

    c. Private communication

    d. Privileged communication

152. The legal term used to describe when a patient has the right to maintain control over certain personal information is referred to as:

    a. Access

    b. Confidentiality

    c. Privacy

    d. Security

153. Who has the legal right to refuse treatment? (Choose all that apply.)

> 1. Juanita, who is 98 years old and of sound mind.
> 2. Christopher, who is 10 years old and of sound mind.
> 3. Jane, who is 35, incompetent, and did not express her treatment wishes prior to becoming incompetent.
> 4. Linda, who is 35, incompetent, and created a Living Will prior to becoming incompetent stating that she did not wish to be kept alive by artificial means.
> 5. William, a 35-year-old born with mental retardation who has the mental capacity of a 12-year-old.

    a. 1 and 2

    b. 1 and 3

    c. 1 and 4

    d. 4 and 5

154. Mrs. Davis is preparing to undergo hernia repair surgery at Deaconess Hospital. Select the best statement of the following options:

    a. An employee from the hospital's surgery department should obtain Mrs. Davis' informed consent.

    b. The surgeon should obtain Mrs. Davis' informed consent.

    c. It does not matter who obtains Mrs. Davis' informed consent as long as it is documented in her medical record.

    d. Informed consent is not necessary because this is not major surgery.

155. Janice arrives at her physician's office for her 10:30 a.m. scheduled appointment and pays her office visit copayment. Her physician examines her. Based on these facts, Janice's consent is:

    a. Informed

    b. Express

    c. Implied

    d. Not necessary

156. St. Joseph's Hospital has a psychiatric service on the sixth floor of the hospital. A 31-year-old male has come to the HIM department and requested to see a copy of his medical record. He has told your clerk he was a patient of Dr. Schmidt, a psychiatrist, and was on the sixth floor of St. Joseph's for the last two months. These records are not psychotherapy notes. The best course of action for you to take, as the HIM director, is:

    a. Prohibit the patient from accessing his record, as it contains psychiatric diagnoses that may greatly upset him.

    b. Allow the patient to access his record.

    c. Allow the patient to access his record if, after contacting his physician, his physician does not feel it will be harmful to the patient.

    d. Deny access because HIPAA prevents patients from reviewing their psychiatric records.

157. Jack Mitchell, a patient in Ross Hospital, is being treated for gallstones. He has not opted out of the facility directory. Callers who request information about him may be given:

    a. No information due to the highly sensitive nature of his illness

    b. Admission date and location in the facility

    c. General condition and acknowledgment of admission

    d. Location in the facility and diagnosis

158. The sequence of the correct steps when evaluating an ethical problem is:

    a. Consider the values and obligations of others; consider the choices that are both justified and not justified; determine the facts; identify prevention options.

    b. Consider the choices that are both justified and not justified; consider the values and obligations of others; identify prevention options; determine the facts.

    c. Determine the facts; consider the choices that are both justified and not justified; consider the values and obligations of others; identify prevention options.

    d. Determine the facts; consider the values and obligations of others; consider the choices that are both justified and not justified; identify prevention options.

159. The Privacy Rule generally requires documentation related to its requirements to be retained:

    a. 3 years

    b. 5 years

    c. 6 years

    d. 10 years

160. Mr. Smith was admitted to University Hospital by Dr. Collins. Mr. Smith's hospital bill will be paid by Blue Cross Insurance. Upon discharge from the hospital, who owns the health record of Mr. Smith?

    a. Mr. Smith

    b. Blue Cross

    c. University Hospital

    d. Dr. Collins

161. Dr. Smith, a member of the medical staff, asks to see the medical records of his adult daughter who was hospitalized in your institution for a tonsillectomy at age 16. The daughter is now 25. Dr. Jones was the patient's physician. Of the options listed here, what is the best course of action?

    a. Allow Dr. Smith to see the records because he was the daughter's guardian at the time of the tonsillectomy.

    b. Call the hospital administrator for authorization to release the record to Dr. Smith since he is on the medical staff.

    c. Inform Dr. Smith that he cannot access his daughter's health record without her signed authorization allowing him access to the record.

    d. Refer Dr. Smith to Dr. Jones and release the record if Dr. Jones agrees.

162. Which of the following laws requires the reporting of deaths and severe complications resulting from the use of medical devices?

    a. Medical Implantation and Transplantation Act of 1986

    b. Medical Devices Reporting Act of 1972

    c. Food and Drug Modernization Act of 1997

    d. Safe Medical Devices Act of 1990

163. Which of the following four sources of law is also known as judge-made or case law?

    a. Constitutional law

    b. Statutory law

    c. Common law

    d. Administrative law

164. Medical information loses PHI status and is no longer protected by the HIPAA Privacy Rule when it:

    a. Becomes an oral communication

    b. Is deidentified

    c. Is used for TPO

    d. Is individually identifiable

165. Linda Wallace is being admitted to the hospital. She is presented with a Notice of Privacy Practices. In the Notice, it is explained that her PHI will be used and disclosed for treatment, payment, and operations (TPO) purposes. Linda states that she does not want her PHI used for those purposes.

    a. The hospital must honor her wishes and not use her PHI for TPO.

    b. The hospital may decline to treat Linda because of her refusal.

    c. The hospital is not required to honor her wishes in this situation, as the Notice of Privacy Practices is informational only.

    d. The hospital is not required to honor her wishes for treatment purposes but must honor them for payment and operations purposes.

166. Sally Mitchell was treated for kidney stones at Graham Hospital last year. She now wants to review her medical record in person. She has requested to review them by herself in a closed room.

    a. Failure to accommodate her wishes will be a violation under the HIPAA Privacy Rule.

    b. Sally owns the information in her record, so she must be granted her request.

    c. Sally's request does not have to be granted because the hospital is responsible for the integrity of the medical record.

    d. Patients should never be given access to their actual medical records.

167. The Kids' Foundation, a foundation related to Children's Hospital, is mailing fundraising information to the families of all patients who have been treated at Children's in the past three years. Based on the facts given:

    a. Children's Hospital violated the privacy rule by giving information to the foundation.

    b. Children's Hospital must have notified the patients/patients' guardians of this disclosure in the Notice of Privacy Practices.

    c. The Kids' Foundation cannot solicit donations from patients' families under any circumstances.

    d. The Kids' Foundation must request authorization from each patient/patient guardian to mail fundraising information out to their families.

168. You are a member of the hospital's Health Information Management Committee. The committee has created a HIPAA-complaint authorization form. Which of the following items does the Privacy Rule require for the form?

    a. Signature of the patient's attending physician

    b. Identification of patient's next of kin

    c. Identification of person/organization authorized to receive PHI

    d. Patient's insurance information

169. Which of the following is an identifier under the Privacy Rule?

    a. Gender

    b. Vehicle license plate

    c. Age

    d. Vital sign recordings

Domain VI   *Legal and Regulatory Standards*

170. Abbreviations can be a source of patient safety issues due to misinterpretation and miscommunication. Abbreviations in the health record:

    a. Are not permitted by Joint Commission standards

    b. Should have only one meaning

    c. Enhance patient safety

    d. Are critical to an electronic health record system

171. Which of the following is a ruling handed down by a court to settle a legal dispute?

    a. Municipal code

    b. Statute

    c. Deemed status

    d. Judicial decision

172. The system that will allow the Centers for Disease Control and Prevention to monitor trends from disease reporting at the local and state level to look for possible bioterrorism incidents is:

    a. National Electronic Infection Surveillance System

    b. National Electronic Disease Surveillance System

    c. National Administrative Notification Disease Agency

    d. National Infection Foundation Surveillance Administration

173. Which of the following is a governmental designation by the state that is necessary for the facility to offer services?

    a. Survey

    b. Licensure

    c. Certification

    d. Accreditation

174. The federal law that directed the Secretary of Health and Human Services to develop healthcare standards governing electronic data interchange and data security is the:

    a. Medicare Act

    b. Prospective Payment Act

    c. Health Insurance Portability and Accountability Act

    d. Social Security Act

175. Most healthcare information standards have been implemented by:

    a. Federal mandate

    b. Consensus

    c. State regulation

    d. Trade association requirement

176. According to Joint Commission Accreditation Standards, which document must be placed in the patient's record before a surgical procedure may be performed?

    a. Admission record

    b. Physician's order

    c. Report of history and physical examination

    d. Discharge summary

177. Long-term, acute-care hospitals must have an agreement with a quality improvement organization (QIO) for periodic review. Which of the following is among the items reviewed?

    a. The medical necessity, reasonableness, and appropriateness of hospital admissions and discharges

    b. Validity of the hospital's diagnostic and marketing information

    c. Quality of the food services furnished in the hospital

    d. Outcome of treatment

178. The Joint Commission currently identifies core measures that provide an indication of a healthcare facility's performance. The core measure data sets include which of the following?

    a. Myocardial infarction, pneumonia, and HIV/AIDS

    b. Pneumonia, asthma care for children, and gastric ulcers

    c. Pneumonia, heart failure, and myocardial infarction

    d. Heart failure, HIV/AIDS, and myocardial infarction

179. A Joint Commission accredited organization must review their formulary annually to ensure a medication's continued:

    a. Safety and dose

    b. Efficiency and efficacy

    c. Efficacy and safety

    d. Dose and efficiency

180. There continues to be a tremendous number of errors in care administration that occur on a daily basis across the country. In response, the Joint Commission and other agencies have established this act and implemented the National Patient Safety Goals to reduce the occurrence of medical errors.

    a. Core Measure Act

    b. Patient Safety and Quality Improvement Act

    c. To Err Is Human Act

    d. Clinical Practice Standards Act

PRACTICE EXAM 2

Domain I *Health Data Management*

1. Mary Smith, RHIA, has been asked to work on the development of a hospital trauma data registry. Which of the following data sets would be most helpful in developing this registry?

   a. DEEDS

   b. UACDS

   c. MDS

   d. OASIS

2. Who owns the health records of patients treated in a healthcare facility?

   a. The patient

   b. The physician

   c. The facility

   d. The patient's family

3. The Preadmission Screening Assessment and Annual Resident Review (PASARR) is a requirement that provides a mechanism for screening mental illness and mental retardation (MI/MR) and is mandated by:

   a. The federal government

   b. State government

   c. Local government

   d. Both the federal and state government

4. This type of data display tool is a plotted chart of data that shows the progress of a process over time.

   a. Bar graph

   b. Histogram

   c. Pie chart

   d. Line graph

5. A coding supervisor audits coded records to ensure the codes reflect the actual documentation in the health record. This process addresses the data quality element of:

   a. Validity

   b. Granularity

   c. Timeliness

   d. Reliability

6. The medical report that documents the response of one member of the medical staff to a request by another member of the medical staff to review a patient's history, examination of the patient, and written findings giving recommendations is:

   a. History and physical exam

   b. Pathology report

   c. Discharge report

   d. Consultation report

7. Which of the following examples illustrates data that have been transformed into meaningful information?

   a. 45%

   b. 3,567 units of penicillin

   c. $5 million

   d. The average length of stay at Holt Hospital is 5.6 days.

8. The processes of retention and destruction of health information are subject to specific regulations in many states as well as guidelines found in federal regulations and _____ standards.

   a. Centers for Medicare and Medicaid

   b. Accreditation

   c. Licensure

   d. HIPAA

9. Copies of personal health records (PHRs) are considered part of the legal health record when:

   a. Consulted by the provider to gain information on a consumer's health history

   b. Used by the organization to provide treatment

   c. Used by the provider to obtain information on a consumer's prescription history

   d. Used by the organization to determine a consumer's DNR status

10. A health record that maintains information throughout the lifespan of the patient, ideally from birth to death, is known as a:

    a. Problem-oriented health record

    b. Patient-centric record

    c. Longitudinal health record

    d. Health record

11. Which of the following statements does not pertain to paper-based health records?

    a. They are kept in locked storage areas that are accessible only to authorized staff.

    b. They are logged out according to the organization's prescribed procedure.

    c. They are forwarded to the appropriate service area when needed for patient care purposes.

    d. They have a built-in access control mechanism.

12. Under which circumstances may an interval note be added to a patient's health record in place of a complete history and physical?

    a. When the patient is readmitted a second time for the same condition

    b. When the patient is readmitted within 30 days of the initial treatment for a different condition

    c. When the patient is readmitted a third time for the same condition

    d. When the patient is readmitted within 30 days of the initial treatment for the same condition

13. The _____ is the procedure that was performed for the definitive treatment (rather than the diagnosis) of the main condition or a complication of the condition.

    a. Chief procedure

    b. Principal treatment

    c. Principal procedure

    d. Comorbidity

14. Who is responsible for writing and signing discharge summaries and discharge instructions?

    a. Attending physician

    b. Head nurse

    c. Primary physician

    d. Admitting nurse

15. The clinical statement: "microscopic sections of the gallbladder reveal a surface lined by tall columnar cells of uniform size and shape" would be documented on which health record form?

    a. Operative report

    b. Pathology report

    c. Discharge summary

    d. Nursing note

16. Today, _____ refers to the level of skilled care needed by patients with complex medical conditions, typically Medicare patients who have multiple medical problems.

    a. Acute care

    b. Ambulatory care

    c. Subacute care

    d. High-quality care

17. Code the following scenario: Patient admitted with major depression, recurrent, severe.

296.30	Major depressive disorder, recurrent episode, unspecified
296.33	Major depressive disorder, recurrent episode, severe, without mention of psychotic behavior
296.89	Other and unspecified bipolar disorders, other
311	Depressive disorder, not elsewhere classified

    a. 296.33

    b. 296.30

    c. 311

    d. 296.89

18. Assign codes for the following scenario: A 35-year-old male is admitted with esophageal reflux. A esophagoscopy and closed esophageal biopsy was performed.

530.10	Esophagitis, unspecified
530.81	Esophageal reflux
530.89	Other specified disorders of esophagus, other
42.23	Other esophagoscopy
42.24	Closed [endoscopic] biopsy of esophagus
45.16	Esophagogastroduodenoscopy [EGD] with closed biopsy

    a. 530.89, 42.24

    b. 530.10, 45.16

    c. 530.81, 42.24

    d. 530.81, 42.23

19. Code the following scenario: Patient with flank pain was admitted and found to have a calculus of the kidney. Ureteroscopy with placement of ureteral stents was performed.

592.0	Calculus of kidney
592.9	Urinary calculus, unspecified
788.0	Renal colic
56.0	Transurethral removal of obstruction from ureter and renal pelvis
59.8	Ureteral catheterization

    a. 592.0, 788.0, 59.8

    b. 788.0, 592.0, 56.0

    c. 592.9, 59.8

    d. 592.0, 59.8

20. Assign codes for the following scenario: A female patient is admitted for stress incontinence. A urethral suspension is performed.

625.6	Stress incontinence female
788.0	Renal colic
788.30	Urinary incontinence, unspecified
57.32	Diagnostic procedure on bladder, other cystoscopy
59.5	Retropubic urethral suspension

    a. 625.6, 57.32

    b. 788.0, 59.5

    c. 625.6, 59.5

    d. 788.30

21. Patient is 47 years old. What is the correct code for an initial inguinal herniorrhaphy for incarcerated hernia?

    a. 49496, Repair, initial inguinal hernia, full-term infant younger than age 6 months, or preterm infant older than 50 weeks postconception age and younger than age 6 months at the time of surgery, with or without hydrocelectomy; incarcerated or strangulated

    b. 49501, Repair initial inguinal hernia, age 6 months to younger than 5 years, with or without hydrocelectomy; incarcerated or strangulated

    c. 49507, Repair initial inguinal hernia, age 5 years or older; incarcerated or strangulated

    d. 49521, Repair recurrent inguinal hernia, any age; incarcerated or strangulated

22. Patient had a laparoscopic incisional herniorrhaphy for a recurrent reducible hernia. The repair included insertion of mesh. What is the correct code assignment?

49560	Repair initial incisional or ventral hernia; reducible
49565	Repair recurrent incisional or ventral hernia; reducible
49568	Implantation of mesh or other prosthesis for open incisional or ventral hernia repair or mesh for closure of debridement for necrotizing soft-tissue infection
49656	Laparoscopy, surgical, repair, recurrent incisional hernia (includes mesh insertion, when performed); reducible

    a. 49565

    b. 49565, 49568

    c. 49656

    d. 49560, 49568

23. What is the correct CPT code assignment for hysteroscopy with lysis of intrauterine adhesions?

58555	Hysteroscopy, diagnostic (separate procedure)
58559	Hysteroscopy, surgical; with lysis of intrauterine adhesions (any method)
58740	Lysis of adhesions (salpingolysis, ovariolysis)

    a. 58555, 58559

    b. 58559

    c. 58559, 58740

    d. 58555, 58559, 58740

24. The physician performs an exploratory laparotomy with bilateral salpingo-oophorectomy. What is the correct CPT code assignment for this procedure?

49000	Exploratory laparotomy, exploratory celiotomy with or without biopsy(s) (separate procedure)	
58700	Salpingectomy, complete or partial, unilateral or bilateral (separate procedure)	
58720	Salpingo-oophorectomy, complete or partial, unilateral or bilateral (separate procedure)	
58940	Oophorectomy, partial or total, unilateral or bilateral	
–50	Bilateral procedure	

    a. 49000, 58940, 58700

    b. 58940, 58720–50

    c. 49000, 58720

    d. 58720

25. Two clerks are abstracting data for a registry. When their work is checked, discrepancies are found between similar data abstracted by the two clerks. Which data quality component is lacking?

    a. Completeness

    b. Validity

    c. Reliability

    d. Timeliness

26. The term "hard coding" refers to:

    a. CPT codes that are coded by the coders

    b. CPT codes that appear in the hospital's Chargemaster

    c. ICD-9-CM codes that are coded by the coders

    d. ICD-9-CM codes that appear in the hospital's Chargemaster

27. Aging of accounts is the practice of counting the days, generally in increments, from the time a bill has been sent to the payer to the current day. What is the standard increment, in days, that most healthcare organizations use for the aging of accounts?

    a. 7-day

    b. 14-day

    c. 30-day

    d. 90-day

28. Most facilities begin counting days in accounts receivable at which of the following times?

    a. Date the patient registers

    b. Date the patient is discharged

    c. Date the bill drops

    d. Date the bill is received by the payer

29. Medicare Part B covers which item(s)?

    a. Eyeglasses and hearing aids

    b. Durable medical equipment

    c. Custodial care

    d. Dentures and dental care

30. Which of the following is the definition of revenue cycle management?

    a. The regularly repeating set of events that produce revenue or income

    b. The method by which patients are grouped together based on a set of characteristics

    c. The systematic comparison of the products, services, and outcomes of one organization with those of a similar organization

    d. Coordination of all administrative and clinical functions that contribute to the capture, management, and collection of patient service revenue

31. The Civilian Health and Medical Program of the Department of Veterans Affairs (CHAMPVA) is available for:

    a. Veterans of the Armed Forces

    b. Spouses or widow(er)s of veterans meeting specific criteria

    c. Active-duty service members

    d. Spouses of active duty service members

32. The physician's office sent a request for payment to Able Insurance Company. The term used in the healthcare industry for this request for payment is a(n):

    a. Allowance

    b. Reimbursement

    c. Block grant

    d. Claim

33. Using the information provided, if this is a participating physician who accepts assignment, how much can he or she expect to be reimbursed by Medicare?

    > Physician's normal charge = $340
    > Medicare fee schedule = $300
    > Patient has met his deductible.

    a. $140

    b. $240

    c. $300

    d. $340

34. Verbal orders by telephone or in person are discouraged. In cases where verbal orders are necessary, which of the following is the most effective method by which the risk of miscommunication can be lessened?

    a. Person receiving the order should read it back to ensure the order is correct.

    b. Order should be signed after the patient is discharged from the facility.

    c. Order should be signed by another provider.

    d. Person receiving the order should authenticate the order after it is entered into the record.

35. Both HEDIS and the Joint Commission's ORYX program are designed to collect data to be used for:

    a. Performance improvement programs

    b. Billing and claims data processing

    c. Developing hospital discharge abstracting systems

    d. Developing individual care plans for residents

36. In data quality management, _____ is the process of translating data into information utilized for an application.

    a. Analysis

    b. Warehousing

    c. Collection

    d. Application

Domain II *Health Statistics and Research Support*

37. The distribution in this curve is:

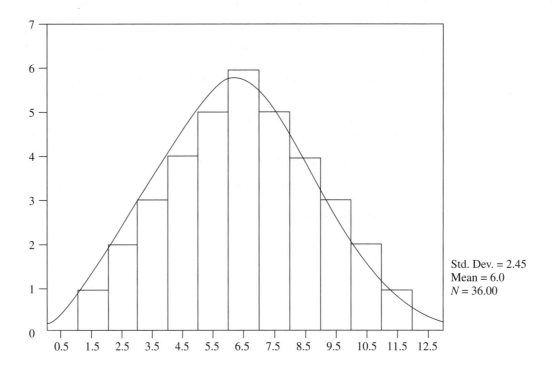

Std. Dev. = 2.45
Mean = 6.0
$N = 36.00$

 a. Normal

 b. Bimodal

 c. Skewed left

 d. Skewed right

38. You want to graph the number of deaths due to prostate cancer from 2000 through 2009. Which graphic tool would you use?

 a. Frequency polygon

 b. Histogram

 c. Line graph

 d. Pie chart

39. In which of the following examples does the gender of the patient constitute information rather than a data element?

 a. As an entry to be completed on the face sheet of the health record

 b. In the note "50-year-old white male" in the patient history

 c. In a study comparing the incidence of myocardial infarctions in black males as compared to white females

 d. In a study of the age distribution of lung cancer patients

40. After evaluating the following graph, what information can be determined from these data?

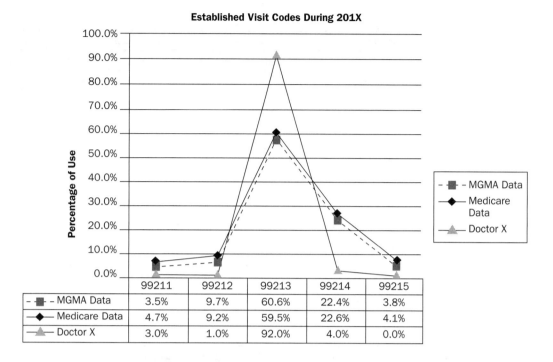

Established Visit Codes During 201X

	99211	99212	99213	99214	99215
- ■ - MGMA Data	3.5%	9.7%	60.6%	22.4%	3.8%
◆ Medicare Data	4.7%	9.2%	59.5%	22.6%	4.1%
▲ Doctor X	3.0%	1.0%	92.0%	4.0%	0.0%

a. Doctor X uses code 99215 less frequently than his peers.

b. Doctor X's documentation doesn't support the codes submitted.

c. Doctor X overutilizes code 99213 as compared with the documentation.

d. Doctor X overutilizes code 99212 as compared with his peers.

41. A hospital is undergoing a major reconstruction project and a new director of nursing has been hired. At the same time, the nursing documentation component of the EHR has been implemented. The fact that nurse staffing satisfaction scores have risen is:

a. A result of anecdotal benefits of EHR

b. A result of qualitative benefits of EHR

c. A result of reconfiguration of the nursing units

d. Uncertain due to existence of confounding variables

42. Using the admission criteria provided, determine if the following patient meets severity of illness and intensity of service criteria for admission.

Severity of Illness	Intensity of Service
Persistent fever	Inpatient-approved surgery/procedure within 24 hours of admission
Active bleeding	Intravenous medications and/or fluid replacement
Wound dehiscence	Vital signs every 2 hours or more often

John Smith presents to the emergency room at 1,500 hours with a fever of 101 degrees F, which he has had for the last three days. He was discharged 6 days ago following a colon resection. X-rays show a bowel obstruction and the plan is to admit him to surgery in the morning.

a. The patient does not meet both severity of illness and intensity of service criteria.

b. The patient does meet both severity of illness and intensity of service criteria.

c. The patient meets intensity of service criteria but not severity of illness.

d. The patient meets severity of illness criteria but not intensity of service.

43. Using the following data, what conclusions can you draw about Dr. Jones' outcomes compared to the OB/GYN practice group?

Category	Dr. Jones	OB/GYN Group
Cesarean section rate	15.2%	11.5%
Hospital-acquired infection	1.7%	1.5%
Surgical wound infection rate	3.8%	0.36%
Mortality rate	0.57%	0.07%

a. Dr. Jones performed better in all four categories than the OB/GYN group.

b. Dr. Jones performed poorer in all four categories than the OB/GYN group.

c. Dr. Jones performed better in all categories except Mortality Rate than the OB/GYN group.

d. Dr. Jones performed poorer in all categories except the Mortality Rate than the OB/GYN group.

44. Using the data in the following graph we can see changes in this hospital profile. What concerns might the hospital's quality council need to address based on these changes in their customer base?

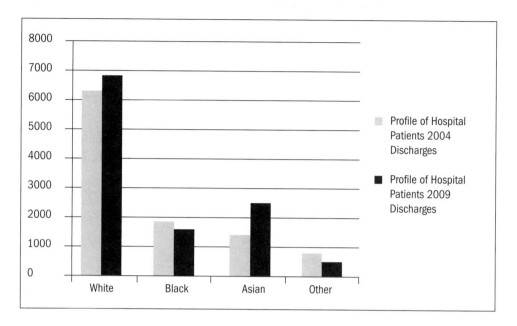

a. Staffing changes might be necessary to accommodate patients who have religious and cultural differences.

b. Data collection has improved.

c. No changes in staffing are necessary because the patient mix is appropriate.

d. The quality council should ask for more detailed data.

45. There were 25 inpatient deaths, including newborns, at Community Memorial Hospital during the month of June. The hospital performed five autopsies during the same period. The gross autopsy rate for the hospital for June was:

a. 0.02%

b. 0.2%

c. 5%

d. 20%

46. Dr. Smith, an OB-GYN specialist, is granted membership on the Medical Center Hospital medical staff, where she may offer care and treatment related to obstetrics and gynecology including performing deliveries and doing gynecological surgery. The process of defining what services she may perform is called:

a. Outcomes management

b. Care mapping

c. Granting privileges

d. Retrospective review

47. James Walker, an 85-year-old male, is admitted with a hip fracture that is repaired with a closed reduction and stabilization. During his hospital stay, a social worker assesses his situation and determines that long-term care placement is necessary when he is ready to leave the hospital. This process is called:

    a. Preadmission review

    b. Continued stay review

    c. Ancillary services review

    d. Discharge planning

48. A risk manager is called in to evaluate a situation in which a visitor to the hospital slipped on spilled water, fell, and fractured his femur. This situation was referred to the risk manager because it involves a:

    a. Medical error

    b. Claims management issue

    c. Potentially compensable event

    d. Sentinel event

49. When the Institute of Medicine and other authors talk about the "quality gap," this can best be described as the:

    a. Time between data analysis and implementation of an improved process

    b. Difference between the patient care protocols belonging to a variety of healthcare providers

    c. Difference between average care and best care

    d. Difference between what is written in a procedure and how the procedure is actually carried out

50. The national association that promotes quality care by certifying qualified professionals is known as the:

    a. National Committee on Quality Assurance

    b. National Association of Healthcare Quality

    c. Institute for Clinical Systems Improvement

    d. Healthcare Facilities Accreditation Program

51. Which of the following is a common resource used in hospitals for the evaluation of outcomes management to improve the clinical performance?

    a. OSHA standards

    b. Core measures

    c. OASIS data set

    d. Marketing plan

52. On his first day of work, the new clerk in release of information processed three requests for information. He observed that all three requests were from law firms. He concluded that all requests for information come from law firms. What type of reasoning did the clerk use?

    a. Clinical

    b. Inductive

    c. Deductive

    d. General

53. The director of the health information department wanted to determine the level of physicians' satisfaction with the departmental services. The director surveyed the physicians who came to the department. What type of sample is this?

    a. Direct

    b. Positive

    c. Guided

    d. Convenience

54. Community Memorial Hospital had 25 inpatient deaths, including newborns, during the month of June. The hospital had a total of 500 discharges for the same period, including deaths of adults, children, and newborns. The hospital's gross death rate for the month of June was:

    a. 0.05%

    b. 2%

    c. 5%

    d. 20%

55. A statewide cancer data system is an example of:

    a. Reference data

    b. Epidemiological data

    c. Coded data

    d. Demographic data

56. Community Memorial Hospital discharged nine patients on April 1st. The length of stay for each patient is shown in the following table. What is the mode length of stay for this group of patients?

Patient	Number of Days
A	1
B	5
C	3
D	3
E	8
F	8
G	8
H	9
I	9

    a. 5 days

    b. 6 days

    c. 8 days

    d. 9 days

Domain III Information Technology and Systems

57. Which one of the following is included in an RFP?

    a. Preparing and training managers

    b. General product information

    c. Establishing an IT infrastructure

    d. A statement describing the criteria to be used in evaluating proposals

58. Which of the following is the first step in a generic approach to developing a strategic IS plan?

    a. Identify the organization's IS needs and prioritize current and future IS projects.

    b. Gain approval from the organization's leaders for the prioritized plan for completing IS projects.

    c. Review the organization's strategic plan and assess the organization's current external and internal environment.

    d. Evaluate the organization's existing information systems and assess its current internal environment.

59. In which stage of the system life cycle would data be collected from system users regarding their needs?

    a Implementation

    b. Design

    c. Analysis

    d. Initiation

60. Which activity would typically occur during the analysis phase of the systems development life cycle (SDLC)?

    a. Researching vendor qualifications

    b. Building interfaces

    c. Definition of functional requirements

    d. Submission of RFI to vendors

61. Which of the following is an effective method of evaluating responses to a request for proposal (RFP)?

    a. Testing the new system

    b. Negotiating contracts with all vendors and assessing the best price

    c. Attending user group meetings

    d. Visiting sites that use the systems of product competitors

62. Which RFP component would fit the following description?

Describe how your product supports the ability to register a patient in the clinic, admit the patient using the same health record number and demographic information, and share medication list for medication reconciliation with the nursing home to which the patient is discharged.

   a. Application support

   b. Operational requirements

   c. Technical specifications

   d. Use case

63. What architectural model of health information exchange allows participants to access data in point-to-point exchange?

   a. Consolidated

   b. Federated—consistent database

   c. Federated—inconsistent databases

   d. Switch

64. Which of the following basic services provided by an HIE organization ensures that information can be retrieved as needed?

   a. Consent management

   b. Person identification

   c. Registry and directory

   d. Secure data transport

65. When an ERD is implemented as a relational database, an entity will become a(n):

   a. Query

   b. Form

   c. Object

   d. Table

66. Which of the following is an example of a 1:1 relationship?

   a. Patients to hospital admissions

   b. Patients to consulting physicians

   c. Patients to clinics

   d. Patients to hospital bed

67. The process of recording representations of human thought, perceptions, or actions in documenting patient care, as well as device-generated information that is gathered and/or computed about a patient as part of healthcare describes:

   a. Patient health records

   b. Information capture

   c. Report generation

   d. Patient safety reports

68. Using the information in these partial attribute lists for the PATIENT, VISIT, and CLINIC columns in a relational database, the attribute PATIENT_MRN is listed in both the PATIENT Entity Attributes and the VISIT Entity Attributes, and CLINIC_ID is listed in both the VISIT Entity Attributes and the CLINIC Entity Attributes. What does the attribute CLINIC_ID represent?

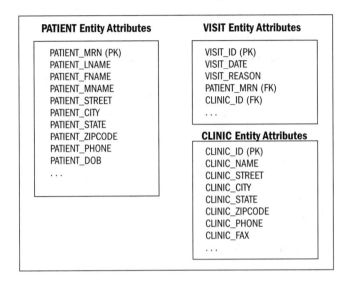

a. It is the foreign key in CLINIC and the primary key in VISIT.

b. It is the primary key in CLINIC and the foreign key in VISIT.

c. It is the primary key in both CLINIC and VISIT.

d. It is the foreign key in both CLINIC and VISIT.

69. What relationships is the following entity relationship diagram showing?

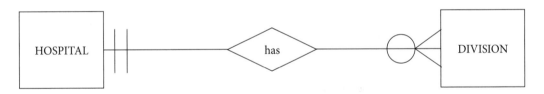

a. Each division has one hospital, but each hospital has many divisions.

b. Each hospital has one division, but each division has many hospitals.

c. Each hospital has one division, and each division has one hospital.

d. Each division has one hospital, and each hospital has one division.

70. A network made accessible to trusted individuals outside of the organization is called a(n):

a. Extranet

b. Intranet

c. VPN

d. LAN

71. Which of the following is a function of a data warehouse?

    a. It provides the most recent transaction data available within the organization.

    b. It stores print-outs from the system in organized files.

    c. It is organized around specific business functions or requirements.

    d. It limits access to business data for analysis or data mining (in other words, decision support).

72. What term is used to refer to an organized collection of data that have been stored electronically to facilitate easy access?

    a. Digital formatting

    b. Database

    c. Telemedicine

    d. Data capture

73. Which of the following health record numbers are in correct terminal digit order?

    a. 00-52-84, 07-48-81, 45-58-81, 65-59-87

    b. 12-25-62, 11-25-68, 18-20-69, 00-24-69

    c. 01-52-25, 02-53-25, 03-22-35, 35-20-35

    d. 00-01-10, 52-01-11, 26-00-00, 00-00-12

74. Dr. Smith orders 500 mg of penicillin by mouth t.i.d. for Jane Doe in the hospital emergency department. The computer sends an alert to Dr. Smith to tell her the patient, Jane Doe, is allergic to penicillin. What type of computer system is Dr. Smith using?

    a. Clinical data repository

    b. Data exchange standard

    c. Clinical decision support

    d. Health informatics standard

75. What process helps to ensure the quality and completeness of health record content in both paper-based and computer-based environments?

    a. Standardization of data-capture tools

    b. Data exchange standards

    c. Standardization of abbreviations

    d. Authentication of health record entries

76. In which EHR database model is all of the organization's patient health information stored in one system?

    a. Distributed

    b. Centralized

    c. Hybrid

    d. Traditional

77. Which of the following would be used to determine what the users need in an information system?

    a. Questionnaire

    b. Trouble ticket

    c. Source code

    d. Weighted system

78. A number assigned to patients in a cancer registry in the order that the patients were entered in the registry every year (for example, 03-0001) is a(n) _____ number.

    a. Accession

    b. Reference

    c. Follow-up

    d. Tracking

79. Which of the following is a systematic process of identifying security measures to afford protections given an organization's specific environment?

    a. Gap analysis

    b. Operations review

    c. Readiness assessment

    d. Risk analysis

80. Which of the following indexes and databases includes patient-identifiable information?

    a. MEDLINE

    b. Clinical trials database

    c. Master population/patient index

    d. UMLS

81. What is the most common type of security threat to a health information system?

    a. External to the organization

    b. Internal to the organization

    c. Environmental in nature

    d. Computer viruses

82. Under what access security mechanism would an individual be allowed access to ePHI if they have proper log-in and password, belong to a specified group, and their workstation is located in a specific place within the facility?

    a. Role-based

    b. User-based

    c. Context-based

    d. Job-based

83. What does entity authentication mean?

    a. Prevents rebooting to deactivate a log-off system

    b. Computer reads a predetermined set of criteria to determine if a user is who he or she claims to be

    c. Allows rebooting to activate a sign-in process

    d. Computer rejects multiple log-ins

84. What is the other term used to denote contingency planning which is a requirement of HIPAA?

    a. Data backup

    b. Data recovery

    c. Disaster recovery planning

    d. Emergency mode of operation

85. Computer-based recognition of handwritten, free-text characters is known as:

    a. Optical character recognition

    b. Intelligent character recognition

    c. Voice recognition

    d. Natural language processing

86. Online/real-time transaction processing (OLTP) is a functional requirement for a:

    a. Data repository

    b. Data mart

    c. Data warehouse

    d. Data dictionary

87. A CT scan is an example of _____ data.

    a. Audio

    b. Bit-mapped

    c. Free-text

    d. Structured

88. Bar coding technology is an example of:

    a. Character/symbol recognition technology

    b. Artificial intelligence

    c. Voice recognition

    d. Vector graphic data

89. In a decision support system, rule-based systems that mimic human thought and enable computers to think in inexact terms are based on:

    a. Fuzzy logic

    b. Genetic algorithms

    c. Symbolic reasoning

    d. Problem analytics

90. Dr. Jones has signed a statement that all of her dictated reports should be automatically considered approved and signed unless she makes corrections within 72 hours of dictating. This is called:

    a. Autoauthentication

    b. Electronic signature

    c. Telecommuting

    d. Chart tracking

91. A system that monitors a patient's cardiac activity and alerts the provider to readings outside normal parameters is an example of a(n):

    a. Point-of-care information system

    b. Clinical pathway

    c. Physiological signal processing system

    d. Telehealth system

92. The MPI includes which of the following information?

    a. Patient's date of birth, height, and gender

    b. Patient's health record number, blood pressure reading, and age

    c. Patient's gender, height, and weight

    d. Patient's date of birth, gender, and health record number

Domain IV *Organization and Management*

93. Outpatient programs designed to provide employees immediate access to psychological counseling on a limited basis and may be provided on-site or through local providers are called:

    a. Employee mental health assistance

    b. Employee assistance programs

    c. Outpatient employee care

    d. Employee crisis lines

94. Which discipline defines the natural laws of work and focuses on employee comfort and safety?

    a. Aesthetics

    b. Cybernetics

    c. Ergonomics

    d. Affinity grouping

95. This process ☐ icon symbol is used in flowcharting to indicate:

    a. A process when actions are being performed by humans

    b. A point in the process at which participants must evaluate the status of the process

    c. Formal procedures that participants are expected to carry out the same way every time

    d. A point in the process where the participants must record data in paper-based or computer-based formats

96. According to the records kept on filing unit performance over the past year, the filing unit has filed an average of 1,000 records per day. You have three FTE record filers in the department who are productive 88 percent of each workday (that is, 12 percent unproductive or 12 percent PFD). Based on this information, the average number of records filed per productive hour per FTE is:

   a. 14 charts/hour

   b. 16 charts/hour

   c. 37 charts/hour

   d. 48 charts/hour

97. Which of the following can be defined as "the planned coordination of the activities of more than one person for the achievement of a common purpose or goal"?

   a. Procedure

   b. Organization

   c. Policy

   d. System

98. A graphic representation of the organization's formal structure is called:

   a. The budget

   b. The mission statement

   c. An organizational chart

   d. Organizational values

99. The following performance standard, "Assign the correct health record number to a returning patient with 99 percent accuracy," is an example of a:

   a. Quality standard

   b. Quantity standard

   c. Joint Commission standard

   d. Compliance standard

100. The following performance standard, "Transcribe 1,500 lines per day," is an example of a:

   a. Quality standard

   b. Quantity standard

   c. Joint Commission standard

   d. Compliance standard

101. What is the usual first step in performance counseling?

   a. Suspension without pay

   b. A demotion

   c. A verbal warning

   d. Conflict resolution

102. What is the focus of conflict management?

    a. Getting personal counseling for the parties involved

    b. Separating the parties involved so that they do not have to work together

    c. Working with the parties involved to find a mutually acceptable solution

    d. Bringing disciplinary action against one party or the other

103. The Hay method is used to measure the three levels of major compensable factors: the know-how, problem-solving, and accountability requirements of each position. This system is used for:

    a. Job evaluation

    b. Interviewing applicants

    c. Performance measurement

    d. Work scheduling

104. A distance learning method where groups of employees in multiple classroom locations may listen to and see the material presented at the same time via satellite or telephone is called:

    a. Audioconferencing

    b. Computer-based training

    c. Teleconferencing

    d. A DVD-ROM

105. Distributing work duties to others along with the right to make decisions and take action is called:

    a. Delegation

    b. Coaching

    c. Accountability

    d. Communication

106. Which is more accurate regarding the role of values in American business?

    a. Most people do not care about the values their organization espouses.

    b. People who believe they work for ethical organizations are more loyal.

    c. The vast majority of people believe their organization operates ethically.

    d. Studies show that values are increasingly unimportant in American business.

107. The *Price Waterhouse v. Hopkins* case was central in showing:

    a. Flawed leaders are widespread across all industries.

    b. Androgenous leadership was more effective than stereotyped leadership.

    c. The glass ceiling no longer operates in American organizations.

    d. Sex discrimination and gender stereotypes were no longer acceptable in organizations.

108. Reductionism refers to the principle that:

    a. Complex processes can be reduced to and analyzed by their independent parts.

    b. A workforce can be downsized without adversely affecting productivity.

    c. Nearly all leadership traits can be reduced to five factors.

    d. The simplest explanation in a theory is generally the best one.

109. Which of the following is an alternate work schedule option that has been made possible by the growth and development of technology?

    a. Compressed workweek

    b. Open systems

    c. Telecommuting

    d. Flextime

110. The accounts receivable collection cycle involves the time from:

    a. Discharge to receipt of the money

    b. Admission to billing the account

    c. Admission to deposit in the bank

    d. Billing of the account to deposit in the bank

111. Of the following, which department is chiefly responsible for capturing the details of a billable event?

    a. Clinical Services

    b. Patient Accounts

    c. Health Information Management

    d. Finance

Use the following information to answer questions 112 through 114.

Triad Healthcare Financial Data 12/31/201X	
Cash	$ 500,000
A/R	$ 250,000
Building	$1,000,000
Land	$ 700,000
A/P	$ 350,000
Mortgage	$ 600,000
Revenue	$2,500,000
Expenses	$2,250,000

112. Based on the financial data listed above, what was Triad's net income?

    a. $150,000

    b. $250,000

    c. $400,000

    d. $1,500,000

113. Based on the financial data listed, what is Triad's total fund balance, *before* posting net income for the year?

    a. $250,000

    b. $400,000

    c. $1,250,000

    d. $1,700,000

114. Based on the financial data listed, what is Triad's total fund balance, *after* posting net income for the year?

    a. $400,000

    b. $1,250,000

    c. $1,500,000

    d. $1,950,000

115. Of the following, which is an example of a contra-account?

    a. Accelerated depreciation

    b. Accumulated depreciation

    c. Depreciation

    d. Historical cost

116. Which of the following are typically required in order to process payment to a vendor?

    a. Invoice, statement, and purchase order

    b. Purchase order, delivery contract, and statement

    c. Receiving document, vendor agreement, and invoice

    d. Purchase order, invoice, shipping, and receiving documents

117. At a cost of $12,000, Community Hospital is refinancing the mortgage on the building that houses its clinic. The hospital will save $500 a month in interest. What is the payback period on the refinancing?

    a. 1 year

    b. 15 months

    c. 18 months

    d. 2 years

118. The primary disadvantage of cost analysis of asset acquisition using payback period is that payback period:

    a. Is difficult to explain to nonfinancial managers

    b. Is difficult to calculate

    c. Ignores the time value of money

    d. Ignores the historical cost of the asset

119. The term _____ represents the significance of a dollar amount based on predetermined criteria.

    a. Variance

    b. Asset

    c. Materiality

    d. Account

120. Contributions to the AHIMA Foundation are deductible as charitable donations as long as no goods or services have been received in return. Therefore, the Foundation is an example of a:

    a. For-profit corporation

    b. Sole proprietorship

    c. Nonprofit corporation

    d. Professional association

121. Using straight-line depreciation, the annual depreciation expense of an item that was purchased for $10,000, had a useful life of 5 years, and a residual value of $500 would be:

    a. $1,500

    b. $1,600

    c. $1,900

    d. $2,000

122. The term _____ represents the totals in accounts (expressed in accounting equation format) at a specific point in time.

    a. Balance sheet

    b. Capital budget

    c. Income statement

    d. Cost report

123. The master list of the individual accounts maintained by an organization is called the:

    a. Journal

    b. Chargemaster

    c. Budget

    d. General ledger

124. Payment of a claim by a third-party payer has which one of the following effects on a hospital's accounts?

    a. It decreases revenue.

    b. It increases accounts receivable.

    c. It increases cash.

    d. It decreases accounts payable.

125. At Community Health Services, each budget cycle provides the opportunity to continue or discontinue services based on available resources so that every department or activity must be justified and prioritized annually in order to effectively allocate resources. Community Health uses what type of operational budget?

   a. Activity-based

   b. Zero-based

   c. Flexible

   d. Fixed

126. Which of the following is the most useful theory for accounting for in-group and out-group formation in the workplace and the role of mentoring?

   a. Vertical Dyad Linkage theory

   b. Contingency theory

   c. Servant leadership

   d. Great Person theory

127. Research on gender and leadership shows that:

   a. There are clear and distinctive differences between men and women in their leadership styles.

   b. There has been little shift in women taking leadership roles in organizations.

   c. Leadership exists in the person, rather than a relationship.

   d. Successful managers are more androgynous.

128. Which of the following is a characteristic of strategic management?

   a. Shifting the balance of power to the employees

   b. Creating a plan to avoid change within the organization

   c. A description of specific implementation plans

   d. A plan to improve the organization's fit with the external world

129. Which of the following best describes the role of strategic management as compared to other management tools and approaches?

   a. A component of each of the major functions of management

   b. An additional function that one learns after mastering other management functions

   c. A replacement for certain management functions

   d. Strategic management has no role with other tools and approaches

130. What is the primary purpose of preparing a vision statement?

   a. To convey a picture of the future

   b. To support a request for an increased budget

   c. To set forth a specific plan of work

   d. To convey a picture of the past

131. Which of the following is most important in securing support for a change program?

    a. Understanding that individuals accept change in their own way

    b. Clear directives from senior management

    c. Assurances that no one will lose his or her job

    d. Being clear about the rewards for those who are on board

132. At Community Memorial Hospital, the coding area has five coders. Each coder is responsible for coding, abstracting, pulling and filing records, answering phones, and maintaining productivity logs. This is an example of _____ work division.

    a. Parallel

    b. Unit

    c. Serial

    d. Serial unit

133. The health information services department at Medical Center Hospital has identified problems with its work processes. Too much time is spent on unimportant tasks, there is duplication of effort, and task assignment is uneven in quality and volume among employees. The manager has each employee complete a form identifying the amount of time he or she spends each day on various tasks. What is this tool called?

    a. Serial work distribution tool

    b. Work distribution chart

    c. Check sheet

    d. Flow process chart

134. When creating work schedules, what is the most important consideration?

    a. All employees work an equal amount of time.

    b. Overtime is avoided.

    c. Float employees cover absences on a daily basis.

    d. Core employees are on duty at times when services must be provided.

135. Work products that must be produced as a result of a project are referred to as:

    a. Materials

    b. Resources

    c. Sponsors

    d. Deliverables

136. As an EHR implementation project proceeds, additional hospital departments add requirements for the system, and the project becomes more complex. This is known as:

    a. Unaligned parameters

    b. Alternative goals

    c. Risk assumption

    d. Scope creep

137. The lead coder in a health information system department has been the acknowledged coding expert for a number of years. As implementation of an encoding system moves forward, it becomes evident this coder has an aversion to technology, is resistant to the encoder, and is losing confidence in her coding skills. In project management terms, this creates a:

    a. Psychological risk

    b. Technical risk

    c. Failure mode

    d. Scope creep

138. A large hospital is planning for an EHR, but wants to ensure it has adequate source systems in place to support it. Each of the ancillary departments has a separate information system and each has claimed that the product is the best on the market and that the vendor has promised the system will interface with any EHR on the market. Identify the project management mistake in this situation.

    a. Lack of priority

    b. Lack of sponsorship

    c. Lack of project manager software

    d. Lack of project management

139. In the following figure, identify the component of the project plan labeled as A.

A				1/12	1/13	1/14	1/15	1/16	1/19	1/20
1.	🖹	1. Test ADT-Lab interface				C				
2.		1.1 Write test scenario	Dr. Smith							
					D		E			
3.	✓ B	1.2 Load test data	John							
4.		1.3 Execute lab order	Mary							

    a. Row numbers

    b. Task completed

    c. Task progress

    d. Dependency

140. An HIM professional who must accurately report HIV status and the true results of an audit that indicates health problems with a local employer, is meeting the ethical standards for:

    a. E-health

    b. Integrated delivery systems

    c. Public health

    d. Managed care

141. What is one reason a risk analysis is performed during the project management process?

    a. The work breakdown structure is hierarchical, not necessarily chronological.

    b. After the initial planning is complete, the plan isn't allowing for potential delays.

    c. The project team members need a list of tasks to perform.

    d. Minor changes to the scope of the project can turn into more significant changes to the original work or cost estimates.

142. An HIM professional who is designing a health record system for a healthcare facility should check _____ to find out how long health records should be retained by the facility.

    a. The attending physician

    b. State and federal law

    c. County or city codes

    d. Joint Commission Accreditation Standards

143. In project management terminology, what is the difference between work and duration?

    a. Work is the amount of effort (usually described in hours) needed to complete the tasks, and the duration is the number of days over which the work will occur.

    b. Work is the amount of effort (usually described in hours) needed to complete the tasks, and the duration is the percentage of the day allotted to work on the task.

    c. Work is the amount of effort (usually described in days) needed to complete the tasks, and the duration is the number of hours over which the work will occur.

    d. There is not a difference; work and duration are the same value.

144. Dr. Blake's administrative assistant purchased office supplies at an office supplies store and charged the purchase to the doctor's account. The journal entry used to record the later payment to the store is a debit to accounts payable and a credit to:

    a. Purchases

    b. Cash

    c. Accounts payable

    d. Revenue

145. What is the strictest measure of an organization's ability to pay its bills on time?

    a. Acid-test ratio

    b. Current ratio

    c. Debt ratio

    d. Accounts receivable ratio

146. Because many employees rate the worst aspect of their job as their immediate supervisor, the base rate for failed leadership can be estimated at:

    a. 10–15%

    b. 25–34%

    c. 42–50%

    d. 65–75%

Domain V *Privacy, Security, and Confidentiality*

147. Which of the following is a rule established by an administrative agency of government?

    a. Municipal code

    b. Statute

    c. Subpoena

    d. Regulation

148. The process of releasing health record documentation originally created by a different provider is called:

    a. Privileged communication

    b. Subpoena

    c. Jurisdiction

    d. Redisclosure

149. What type of health record policy dictates how long individual health records must remain available for authorized use?

    a. Disclosure policies

    b. Legal policies

    c. Retention policies

    d. Redisclosure policies

150. Under the HIPAA privacy standard, which of the following types of protected health information (PHI) must be specifically identified in an authorization?

    a. History and physical reports

    b. Operative reports

    c. Consultation reports

    d. Psychotherapy notes

151. Joe Smith, RHIA, works for an outsourcing company as interim HIS department director in a large hospital. By the terms of the contract, the hospital pays the company for Joe's services based on a 40-hour workweek with overtime for any hours exceeding 40. Joe typically works 9 hours per day, Monday through Thursday, and 4 hours on Friday. He then flies home for the weekend. After several months, he discovers the hospital is billed for 44 to 48 hours per week almost every week. Joe confronts the company billing department because this practice conflicts with the tenet of the AHIMA Code of Ethics that states that health information management professionals:

    a. Respect the rights and dignity of all individuals

    b. Adhere to the vision, mission, and values of the association

    c. Promote and protect the confidentiality and security of health records and health information

    d. Refuse to participate in or conceal unethical practices or procedures

152. What penalties can be enforced against a person or entity that willfully and knowingly violates the HIPAA Privacy Rule with the intent to sell, transfer, or use PHI for commercial advantage, personal gain, or malicious harm?

    a. A fine of not more than $10,000 only

    b. A fine of not more than $10,000, not more than 1 year in jail, or both

    c. A fine of not more than $5,000 only

    d. A fine of not more than $250,000, not more than 10 years in jail, or both

153. Mary is contemplating triple bypass surgery. Informed consent by her surgeon would typically contain which one of the following?

    a. Guarantees for outcomes

    b. Risks associated with the procedure

    c. Insurance coverage for the procedure

    d. Right to access health record of treatment

154. The Patient Self-Determination Act requires healthcare providers to:

    a. Inform patients of their right to create advance directives

    b. Document the presence or absence of an advance directive in a patient's health record

    c. Write advance directives for patients who do not have them

    d. Inform patients of their right to create advance directives and document the presence or absence of an advance directive in a patient's health record

155. Regarding life-sustaining treatment and a patient's right of self-determination, courts have generally held that:

    a. A competent adult does not have the right to refuse medical treatment.

    b. A competent adult gives up the right to refuse medical treatment if the physician believes the refusal is morally wrong.

    c. An incompetent adult has a right to the withdrawal of medical treatment if that incompetent adult, while competent, expressed his/her wishes and the state now determines that the evidence of those wishes is sufficient.

    d. A competent adult cannot make healthcare decisions based on his or her religious beliefs.

156. Johnny is 12 years old and his parents are divorced. In order for Johnny to receive medical treatment, generally:

    a. Both parents must consent

    b. One parent must consent

    c. A court-appointed guardian must consent

    d. Johnny can consent

157. The medical staff at Regency Health is nationally renowned for its skill in performing cardiac procedures. The nursing staff in the cardiac unit has noticed a significant lack of informed consents prior to the performance of procedures. Obtaining informed consent is the responsibility of the:

    a. Nursing staff

    b. Admissions department

    c. Physician

    d. Administration

158. Legally, which of the following is most important in determining the length of time a hospital must retain health records?

    a. Research needs

    b. Storage capabilities

    c. Statute of limitations

    d. Cost

159. Today, Janet Kim visited her new dentist for an appointment. She was not presented with a Notice of Privacy Practices. Is this acceptable?

    a. No; a dentist is a healthcare clearinghouse, which is a covered entity under HIPAA.

    b. Yes; a dentist is not a covered entity per the HIPAA Privacy Rule.

    c. No; it is a violation of the HIPAA Privacy Rule.

    d. Yes; the Notice of Privacy Practices is not required.

160. Mercy Hospital personnel need to review the health records of Katie Grace for utilization review purposes (#1). They will also be sending her records to her physician for continuity of care (#2). Under HIPAA, these two functions are:

    a. Use (#1) and disclosure (#2)

    b. Request (#1) and disclosure (#2)

    c. Disclosure (#1) and use (#2)

    d. Disclosures (#1 and #2)

161. Per the HIPAA Privacy Rule, which of the following requires authorization for research purposes?

    a. Use of Mary's information about her myocardial infarction, deidentified

    b. Use of Mary's information about her asthma, in a limited data set

    c. Use of Mary's individually identifiable information related to her asthma treatments

    d. Use of medical information about Jim, Mary's deceased husband

162. The "custodian of health records" refers to the individual within an organization who is responsible for which one of the following actions?

    a. Authorized to determine alternative treatment for the patient

    b. Prepares physicians to testify

    c. Testifies to authenticity of records

    d. Testifies regarding the care of the patient

163. Under HIPAA, which of the following is named as a covered entity?

    a. Outsourced transcription company

    b. EHR vendor

    c. Healthcare clearinghouse

    d. The patient

164. Shirley Denton has written to request an amendment of her PHI from Bon Voyage Hospital, stating that incorrect information is present on the document in question. The document is an incident report from Bon Voyage Hospital, which was erroneously placed in Ms. Denton's health record. The covered entity declines to grant her request based on which Privacy Rule provision?

    a. It was not created by the covered entity.

    b. It is not part of the designated record set.

    c. None, the covered entity must grant her request.

    d. Her attending physician did not authorize the amendment.

165. Champion Hospital retains Hall and Hall, a law firm, to perform all of its legal work, including representation during medical malpractice lawsuits. Which of the following statements is correct?

    a. The law firm is not a business associate because it is a legal, not a medical, organization.

    b. The law firm is a business associate because it performs activities on behalf of the hospital.

    c. The law firm is not a business associate because the privacy rule prohibits it from using individually identifiable information.

    d. The law firm is not a business associate because it is a medical, not a legal, organization.

166. One of the medical staff committees at St. Vincent Hospital is responsible for reviewing cases of patients readmitted within 14 days after discharge. This review of the patients' health records is considered healthcare:

    a. Actions

    b. Operations

    c. Payment

    d. Treatment

167. Susan is completing her required high school community service hours by serving as a volunteer at the local hospital. Relative to the hospital, Susan is a(n):

    a. Business associate

    b. Employee

    c. Workforce member

    d. Covered entity

168. Jeremy Lykins was required to undergo a physical exam prior to becoming employed by San Fernando Hospital. Jeremy's medical information is:

    a. Protected by the Privacy Rule because it is individually identifiable

    b. Not protected by the Privacy Rule because it is part of a personnel record

    c. Protected by the Privacy Rule because it contains his physical exam results

    d. Protected by the Privacy Rule because it is in the custody of a covered entity

169. Jake Mitchell, a patient in Ross Hospital, is being treated for gallstones. He has not opted out of the facility directory. Callers who request information about him may be given:

    a. No information due to the highly sensitive nature of his illness

    b. Admission date and location in the facility

    c. General condition and acknowledgment of admission

    d. Location in the facility and diagnosis

Domain VI *Legal and Regulatory Standards*

170. During the voluntary review process, the performance of a healthcare organization is measured against:

    a. Accreditation standards

    b. Clinical practice guidelines

    c. Core measures

    d. Conditions of Participation

171. The discharge summary must be completed within _____ after discharge for most patients but within _____ for patients transferred to other facilities. Discharge summaries are not always required for patients who were hospitalized for less than _____ hours.

    a. 30 days/48 hours/24 hours

    b. 14 days/24 hours/48 hours

    c. 14 days/48 hours/24 hours

    d. 30 days/24 hours/48 hours

172. The Patient Self-Determination Act (PSDA 1991) requires healthcare facilities to provide written information on a patient's right to execute this:

    a. Advance directive

    b. Leave the facility against medical advice (AMA)

    c. Choice of physician

    d. Option for autopsy report

173. One technical function that is often the focus of individuals with an associate-level education in the HIM field is abstracting. Abstracting is defined as:

    a. Compiling the pertinent information from the health record based on predetermined data sets

    b. Assigning the appropriate code or nomenclature term for categorization

    c. Assembling a chronological set of data for an express purpose

    d. Conducting qualitative and quantitative analysis of documentation against standards and policy

174. CMS and the Joint Commission both require that healthcare professionals assess the work of colleagues in the same profession; this process is known as:

a. Peer review

b. Utilization review

c. Workflow process

d. Mediation

175. Which of the following is a widely accepted accrediting body for behavioral healthcare organizations?

a. American Psychological Association (APA)

b. Agency for Healthcare Research and Quality (AHRQ)

c. Commission on Accreditation of Rehabilitation Facilities (CARF)

d. National Committee for Healthcare Assurance (NCHA)

176. What type of standard establishes methods for creating unique designations for individual patients, healthcare professionals, healthcare provider organizations, and healthcare vendors and suppliers?

a. Vocabulary standard

b. Identifier standard

c. Structure and content standard

d. Security standard

177. What type of organization works under contract with the CMS to conduct Medicare/Medicaid certification surveys for hospitals?

a. Accreditation organizations

b. Certification organizations

c. State licensure agencies

d. Conditions of Participation agencies

178. What type of standard establishes uniform definitions for clinical terms?

a. Identifier standard

b. Vocabulary standard

c. Transaction and messaging standard

d. Structure and content standard

179. HIPAA mandated that healthcare business partners and covered entities implement a common standard for data and information transfer. That standard is:

a. ICD-9-CM

b. HL7

c. ASC X12 N

d. CPT

180. An advance directive is used to direct an individual's healthcare wishes in the event of:

    a. Surgery

    b. Patient incapacitation

    c. Patient indecisiveness

    d. A disagreement between patient and family

Answer
Key

RHIA

Practice Questions

1. **b** Objective descriptions of processes, procedures, people, and other observable objects and activities are all considered data (Odom-Wesley et al. 2009, 39).

2. **d** Biomedical research is considered an ancillary function of the health record (Odom-Wesley et al. 2009, 46).

3. **c** Clinical practice guidelines are used in reference to electronically accessed information that provides physicians with pertinent health information beyond the health record itself (Odom-Wesley et al. 2009, 124).

4. **b** Hospital vital statistics are reported to the National Vital Statistics System (Odom-Wesley et al. 2009, 58).

5. **b** Patient-focused care attempts to contain hospital inpatient costs and improve quality by restructuring services so that more of them take place in nursing units (patient floors) and not in specialized units in dispersed hospital locations. The emphasis is on cross-training in the nursing units to perform a variety of functions for a small group of patients rather than one set of functions for a large number of patients (LaTour and Eichenwald Maki 2010, 34).

6. **d** The American Medical Association (AMA) was established in 1847, to represent the interests of physicians across the United States. However, the AMA was dominated by members who had strong ties to the medical schools and the status quo. Its ability to lead a reform of the profession was limited until it broke its ties with the medical schools in 1874. At that time, the association encouraged the creation of independent state licensing boards (LaTour and Eichenwald Maki 2010, 9).

7. **d** A license is required in order for medical students to practice medicine (LaTour and Eichenwald Maki 2010, 9).

8. **a** Adoption of the Minimum Standards was the basis of the Hospital Standardization Program and marked the beginning of the modern accreditation process for healthcare organizations. Basically, accreditation standards are developed to reflect reasonable quality standards (LaTour and Eichenwald Maki 2010, 11).

9. **d** Credentialing is the process that requires the verification of the educational qualifications, licensure status, and other experience of healthcare professionals who have applied for the privilege of practicing within a healthcare facility (Odom-Wesley et al. 2009, 52).

10. **b** Audit controls are the mechanisms that record and examine activity in information systems. HIPAA does not specify what form of audit controls must be used, how or how often they must be examined, or how long they must be retained (LaTour and Eichenwald Maki 2010, 255).

11. **b** Quantitative analysis is a review of the health record for identifying deficiencies for completeness and accuracy. It is generally conducted retrospectively, that is, after the patient's discharge from the facility or at the conclusion of treatment (LaTour and Eichenwald Maki 2010, 212).

12. **a** LOINC is a well-accepted set of terminology standards that provide a standard set of universal names and codes for identifying individual laboratory and clinical results. It is managed by the Regenstrief Institute in Indianapolis and was developed using a semantic data model. LOINC codes are widely acceptable and included in the consolidated health informatics standards. LOINC vocabulary is maintained as a single table structure; the database and supporting materials are available for download (LaTour and Eichenwald Maki 2010, 181).

13. **b** The Uniform Ambulatory Care Data Set (UACDS) includes data elements specific to ambulatory care such as the reason for the encounter with the healthcare provider (LaTour and Eichenwald Maki 2010, 166).

14. **b** Medicare requires that all inpatient hospitals collect a minimum set of patient-specific data elements, which are in databases formulated from hospital discharge abstract systems. The patient-specific data elements are referred to as the Uniform Hospital Discharge Data Set (LaTour and Eichenwald Maki 2010, 165–166).

15. **a** X12N refers to standards adopted for electronic data interchange. In order for transmission of healthcare data between a provider and payer, both parties must adhere to these standards (LaTour and Eichenwald Maki 2010, 180–181).

16. **b** Care plans are required documentation in an LTCH. Some LTCHs may use critical paths (or clinical pathways) for specific patients (Odom-Wesley et al. 2009, 357).

17. **b** The content of the Resident Assessment Instruments (RAIs) is ultimately determined by each state and may differ from state to state. The RAI consists of a standard Minimum Data Set, Resident Assessment Protocol, and utilization guidelines (Odom-Wesley et al. 2009, 368).

18. **b** Because of the risks associated with miscommunication, verbal orders are discouraged. When a verbal order is necessary, a clinician should sign, give his or her credential (for example, RN, PT, or LPN), and record the date and time the order was received. Verbal orders for medication are usually required to be given to, and to be accepted only by, nursing or pharmacy personnel (Brodnik et al. 2012, 172).

19. **c** The provider is responsible for ensuring the quality of the documentation of the healthcare record (Brodnik et al. 2012, 169–170).

20. **d** In physician practices, patients are informed of their option to transfer their records to another provider. The majority of complete contracts specify that health records are owned by the provider group (Brodnik et al. 2012, 193).

21. **a** EHR format is arranged in chronological order with documentation from various sources intermingled (Odom-Wesley et al. 2009, 217).

22. **a** Documentation of staff disagreements in the health records heightens the risk of liability for both the healthcare organization and those involved in the disagreement. Individuals documenting in the health record should avoid recording disagreements in the patient record so as not to raise red flags that will result in the record becoming the centerpiece of litigation (Brodnik et al. 2012, 173).

23. **b** When entries are made in the health record regarding a patient who is particularly hostile or irritable, general documentation principles apply, such as charting objective facts and avoiding the use of personal opinions, particularly those that are critical of the patient. The degree to which these general principles apply is heightened because a disagreeable patient may cause a provider to use more expressive and inappropriate language. Further, a hostile patient may be more likely to file legal action in the future if the hostility is a personal attribute and not simply a manifestation of his or her medical condition (Brodnik et al. 2012, 173).

24. **b** Every long-term care facility must complete a comprehensive assessment of every resident's needs by using the Resident Assessment Instrument (RAI) specified by the state in which the facility operates (Odom-Wesley et al. 2009, 368).

25. **b** Natural Language Processing (NLP) uses a technology based on artificial intelligence that extracts pertinent data and terms from a text-based document and converts them into medical codes. The natural language processing technology used might be algorithmic (rules-based) or statistical (LaTour and Eichenwald Maki 2010, 400).

26. **c** Computer-assisted coding (CAC) cannot address the major obstacle facing today's human coder: the lack of accurate, complete clinical documentation (LaTour and Eichenwald Maki 2010, 401).

27. **c** According to the UHDDS definition, ethnicity should be recorded on a patient record as non-Spanish/Hispanic or Spanish/non-Hispanic, or unknown. The UHDDS has been revised several times since 1986 (LaTour and Eichenwald Maki 2010, 166–167).

28. **d** The quality of coded clinical data depends on a number of factors, including reliability. Reliability is the extent to which the data can be reproduced by subsequent measurements or tests (for example, coded clinical data are considered reliable when multiple coders assign the same codes to a record) (LaTour and Eichenwald Maki 2010, 399).

29. **a** Continuity of care record (CCR) is documentation of care delivery from one healthcare experience to another (LaTour and Eichenwald Maki 2010, 178–179).

30. **a** Health Plan Employer Data and Information Set (HEDIS) is a set of standard performance measures designed to provide purchasers and consumers of healthcare with the information they need for comparing the performance of managed healthcare plans (LaTour and Eichenwald Maki 2010, 170).

31. **c** Changes and updates to ICD-9-CM are managed by the ICD-9-CM Coordination and Maintenance Committee, a federal committee co-chaired by representatives from the NCHS and the Centers for Medicare and Medicaid Services (CMS). The NCHS is responsible for Volumes 1 and 2 (Diagnoses), and the CMS is responsible for Volume 3 (Procedures). (LaTour and Eichenwald Maki 2010, 349).

32. **a** An encoder is used to increase the accuracy and efficiency of the coding process. Although encoders can cite official coding guidelines and provide code optimization guidance, they require user interaction. Encoders promote accuracy as well as consistency in the coding of diagnoses and procedures (LaTour and Eichenwald Maki 2010, 400).

33. **d** If the diagnosis documented at the time of discharge is qualified as "probable," "suspected," "likely," "questionable," "possible," or "still to be ruled out," or other similar terms indicating uncertainty, code the condition as if it existed or was established (Schraffenberger 2012, 72).

34. **c** Patients who are admitted for an HIV-related illness should be assigned a minimum of two codes in the following order: code 042 to identify the HIV disease and additional codes to identify the related diagnosis (Schraffenberger 2012, 83–84).

35. **b** Septicemia generally refers to a systemic disease associated with the presence of pathological microorganisms or toxins in the blood, which can include bacteria, viruses, fungi, or other organisms. Code 038.11 is for septicemia with *Staphylococcus aureus*. Because abdominal pain is a symptom of diverticulitis, only the diverticulitis of the colon is coded (Schraffenberger 2012, 80–81).

36. **d** To assign these codes, documentation in the health record must support his causal relationship. When a causal relationship exists, the principal diagnosis code assigned is a diabetic code from category 250, followed by the code for the manifestation or complication. The diabetes codes and the secondary codes that correspond to them are paired codes that follow the etiology/manifestation convention of the classification (Schraffenberger 2012, 124).

37. **c** If the primary malignant neoplasm previously removed by surgery or eradicated by radiotherapy or chemotherapy recurs, the primary malignant code for the site is assigned, unless the Alphabetic Index directs otherwise (Schraffenberger 2012, 106).

38. **a** The repair of the hernia is not coded because it was not performed; however, code 54.19 is assigned to describe the extent of the procedure. The V64.1 is also used to indicate the cancelled procedure due to the contraindication. The code 427.89 is also added for the bradycardia that the patient developed during the procedure (Schraffenberger 2012, 46–47).

39. **b** V codes are diagnosis codes and indicate a reason for a healthcare encounter (Schraffenberger 2012, 432).

40. **b** The fracture is the principal diagnosis, with contusions is a secondary diagnosis. The fracture is what required the most treatment. Procedures for the reduction, debridement, and external fixation device would all need to be coded (Schraffenberger 2012, 66–67, Appendix I).

41. **d** Begin with the main term Revision; pacemaker site; chest (Kuehn 2012, 20, 27).

42. **b** Begin with the main term biopsy, artery, temporal (Kuehn 2012, 20, 27).

43. **a** Code 54401 is correct because the prosthesis is self-contained (Kuehn 2012, 20, 27).

44. **d** Modifier –24 is used for unrelated evaluation and management service by the same physician during a postoperative period (Kuehn 2012, 53).

45. **d** Coverage differs among these states because Medicaid allows states to maintain a unique program adapted to state residents' needs and average incomes. Although state programs must meet coverage requirements for groups such as recipients of adoption assistance and foster care, other types of coverage, such as vision and dental services, are determined by the states' Medicaid agencies (Casto and Layman 2011, 85–86).

46. **a** TRICARE Prime is also available for military retirees under age 65 and their families (Casto and Layman 2011, 88–89).

47. **c**   Each RBRVU comprises three elements, physician work, physician practice expense, and malpractice, each of which is a national average available in the *Federal Register* (Casto and Layman 2011, 152).

48. **a**   Case-mix index is the average of the sum of the relative weights of all patients treated during a specified time period (Casto and Layman 2011, 119).

49. **a**   In the global payment method, the third-party payer makes one combined payment to cover the services of multiple providers who are treating a single episode of care. This payment method consolidates payments from the healthcare payer (Casto and Layman 2011, 11).

50. **b**   Both the MS-LTC-DRGs and the acute care MS-DRGs are based on the principal diagnosis in terms of grouping and reimbursement (Casto and Layman 2011, 211–213).

51. **a**   In the long-term care prospective payment system (LTCH PPS), the standard federal rate is the national base payment amount in the prospective payment system for long-term care hospitals (PPS for LTC) (Casto and Layman 2011, 211).

52. **a**   To meet the CMS's definition of an IRF, facilities must have an inpatient population in which at least 75 percent of the patients require intensive rehabilitation services and one of the 13 conditions: stroke, spinal cord injury, congenital deformity, amputation, major multiple trauma, fracture of femur, brain injury, neurological disorders, burns, active polyarticular rheumatoid arthritis, systemic vasculitides, severe or advanced osteo-arthritis, or knee replacement (Casto and Layman 2011, 215).

53. **a**   The conversion factor is the national dollar multiplier that sets the allowance for the relative values—a constant (Casto and Layman 2011, 154).

54. **c**   Under the HHPPS, CMS has accounted for nonroutine medical supplies, home health aide visits, medical social services, and nursing and therapy services (Casto and Layman 2011, 235).

55. **d**   Under the Medicare hospital outpatient prospective payment system (HOPPS), outpatient services such as recovery room, supplies (other than pass-through), and anesthesia are included in this reimbursement method (Casto and Layman 2011, 178).

56. **d**   Ambulatory payment classifications (APCs) are based on the CPT or HCPCS code(s) reported in billing (Casto and Layman 2011, 177).

57. **a**   An outlier payment is paid when the cost of the service is greater than the APC payment by a fixed ratio and exceeds the APC payment plus a threshold amount (Casto and Layman 2011, 186).

58. **b**   The ambulatory patient groups (APGs) have been adopted for use by many third-party payers for reimbursement in the prospective payment system (Casto and Layman 2011, 174).

59. **a**   The Omnibus Budget Reconciliation Act of 1980 amended sections 1832(a)(2) and 1833 of the Social Security Act (SSA) to specify procedures that would be covered under the prospective payment system called the ASC List of Covered Procedures (ASC list) (Casto and Layman 2011, 187).

60. **d**   Gunshot wounds, physical abuse, and substance abuse are not hospital-acquired conditions and therefore are not listed under the hospital-acquired conditions provision list (Casto and Layman 2011, 283–284).

61. **d**   The Medicare reimbursement for LTCHs is under a PPS based on the Medicare Severity diagnosis-related groups (MS-DRGs) system used by short-term, acute-care hospitals and referred to as MS-LTC-DRGs. The same short-term, acute-care MS-DRGs are used, but have been weighted to reflect the resources required to treat the medically complex patients treated at LTCHs (Casto and Layman 2011, 208).

62. **b**   Fraud is a false representation of fact or a failure to disclose a fact that is material (relevant) to a healthcare transaction that results in damage to another party that reasonably relies on the misrepresentation or failure to disclose (Brodnik et al. 2012, 430).

63. **d**   The Federal Anti-Kickback Statute establishes criminal penalties for individuals and entities that knowingly and willfully offer, pay, solicit, or receive remuneration in order to induce business for which payment may be made under any federal healthcare program. This includes transfer of anything of value, in cash or in kind, whether made directly or indirectly (Brodnik et al. 2012, 435).

64. **c**   Safe harbors are activities that are not subject to prosecution and protect the organization from civil or criminal penalties under the Federal Anti-Kickback Statute. The OIG has created a number of regulatory safe harbors covering such arrangements (Brodnik et al. 2012, 436–437).

65. **d**   The Stark Law or Federal Physician Self-Referral Statute prohibits physicians ordering services for Medicare patients from entities with which the physician or an immediate family member has a financial relationship (Brodnik et al. 2012, 438–439).

66. **c**   Failure to document medical necessity appropriately is one of the two areas in which the OIG says is responsible for 70 percent of bad claims. The other area is insufficient or missing documentation (Brodnik et al. 2012, 438–439).

67. **a**   Packaging means that payment for that service is packaged into payment for other services and, therefore, there is no separate PAC payment. Packaged services might include minor ancillary services, inexpensive drugs, medical supplies, and implantable devices (LaTour and Eichenwald Maki 2010, 393).

68. **c**   Managed care is a generic term for a healthcare reimbursement system that manages cost, quality, and access to services. Most managed care plans do not provide healthcare directly. Instead, they enter into service contracts with the physicians, hospitals, and other healthcare providers who provide medical services to enrollees in the plans (LaTour and Eichenwald Maki 2010, 34).

69. **c**   The adjustment component is called the Geographic Practice Cost Index (GPCI). This index is based on relative differences in the cost of a market basket of goods across geographic areas (Casto and Layman 2011, 167).

70. **a**   Nonparticipating providers (nonPARs) do not sign a participation agreement with Medicare but may or may not accept assignment. If the nonPAR physician elects to accept assignment, he or she is paid 95 percent (5 percent less than participating physicians) of the Medicare fee schedule (MFS). For example, if the MFS amount is $200, the PAR provider receives $160 (80 percent of $200), but the nonPAR provider receives only $152 (95 percent of $160). In this case the physician is Nonparticipating so he/she will receive 95 percent of the 80 percent of the MFS or 80 percent of 300 is $240; 95 percent of the $240 is $228. Medicare will reimburse the physician $240 and the patient's liability is $60 (LaTour and Eichenwald Maki 2010, 405–407).

71. **c**   The subscriber of the insurance policy is the member or person for which the policy is provided for (Casto and Layman 2011, 64).

72. **a**   The policy information provided states this is a single policy or employee-only policy, so the member's spouse is not covered (Casto and Layman 2011, 64).

73. **d**   The third-party payer is not Medicare, Medicaid, or Blue Cross/Blue Shield so it is considered a commercial healthcare insurance company (Casto and Layman 2011, 6).

74. **c**   The policy information provided states this is an employee-only or individual policy so the dependents of Jane E. White would not be covered (Casto and Layman 2011, 64).

75. **b**   The insured is the organization that has purchased the insurance policy. In this case, STATE has purchased the insurance coverage for subscriber Jane B. White (Casto and Layman 2011, 60–61).

76. **d**   The International Organization for Standardization (ISO) is an example of the drive toward quality improvement. This nongovernmental global organization, established in 1987, provides more than 17,000 quality standards for nearly every business, technology, and industry sector. Adopted by more than 157 countries, the generic standards can be applied to organizations of any size. It involves defining, executing, and auditing best practices in production or service delivery (LaTour and Eichenwald Maki 2010, 629).

77. **a**   Vital records are those concerned with births, deaths, marriages, divorces, abortions, and late fetal deaths. In the United States, states require that certificates be completed verifying the vital event (Brodnik et al. 2012, 378).

78. **a**   In 1974, the federal government adopted the UHDDS as the standard for collecting data for the Medicare and Medicaid programs. When the Prospective Payment Act was enacted in 1983, UHDDS definitions were incorporated into the rules and regulations for implementing diagnosis-related groups (DRGs). A key component was the incorporation of the definitions of principal diagnosis, principal procedure, and other significant procedures, into the DRG algorithms (LaTour and Eichenwald Maki 2010, 166).

79. **d**   Source-oriented is a system of health record organization in which information is arranged according to the patient care department that provided the care (LaTour and Eichenwald Maki 2010, 204).

80. **b**   The medical staff is governed by bylaws that are typically voted on by the medical staff and executive committee and then approved by the facility's board (Brodnik et al. 2012, 463).

81. **d**   The medical staff is governed by bylaws that are typically voted on by the medical staff and executive committee and then approved by the facility's board. The organized medical staff operates under the direction of the medical staff officers. The medical staff officers typically consist of a president, president-elect, chief of staff, and vice chief of staff with the president-elect transitioning to president and the vice chief of staff transitioning to the chief of staff position (Brodnik et al. 2012, 464).

82. **b**   The six classification categories of medical staff membership are as follows: active (regular), associate, courtesy, consulting, honorary, and affiliate. The honorary classification category is intended for those medical staff who practice very little and may not admit patients, but their reputation and previous service to the hospital is such that the hospital wants to recognize their contribution (Brodnik et al. 2012, 466).

83. **b**   In order to practice medicine, a physician must graduate from an approved medical school and pass a state-based licensure exam. This exam allows a physician to obtain a drug enforcement agency (DEA) number, required to prescribe medications and practice medicine (Shaw and Elliott 2012, 294–295).

84. **b**   The third key process of data quality management is warehousing, which includes the processes and systems used to archive data and data journals (Odom-Wesley et al. 2009, 257).

85. **a**   Common characteristics of data quality are relevancy, granularity, timeliness, currency, accuracy, precision, and consistency (LaTour and Eichenwald Maki 2010, 119–122).

86. **d**   A fetal death refers to the death of a fetus of a particular weight or gestation frequently 500 g or more or 22 or more completed weeks of gestation (Brodnik et al. 2012, 382).

87. **b**   State laws have developed requirements for certain deaths, such as accidental, homicidal, suicidal, sudden, and suspicious in nature to be reported, usually to the medical examiner or coroner. In addition, deaths as a result of abortion or induced termination of pregnancy are also reportable (Brodnik et al. 2012, 381).

88. **d**   A medical examiner is typically a physician with pathology training given the responsibility by a government, such as a county or state, for investigating suspicious deaths. A coroner is typically an appointed or elected official, who may or may not be a physician, with responsibility for investigating suspicious deaths (Brodnik et al. 2012, 381).

89. **c**   Precision often relates to numerical data. It denotes how close to an actual size, weight, or other standard a particular measurement is (LaTour and Eichenwald Maki 2010, 119).

90. **b**   Data granularity is sometimes referred to as data "atomicity," which means that the individual data elements cannot be further subdivided; they are "atomic" (LaTour and Eichenwald Maki 2010, 119).

91. **b**   The Tax Relief and Health Care Act of 2006 (MIEA-TRHCA) expanded CMS quality initiatives to the hospital outpatient and ambulatory surgical center areas (Casto and Layman 2011, 281).

92. **d**   Secondary analysis is the analysis of the original work of others. In secondary analysis, researchers reanalyze original data by combining data sets to answer new questions or by using more sophisticated statistical techniques. The work of others created the MEDPAR file (LaTour and Eichenwald Maki 2010, 483).

93. **a** The prevalence rate is the proportion of persons in a population who have a particular disease at a specific point in time or over a specified period of time. The prevalence rate describes the magnitude of an epidemic and can be an indicator of the medical resources needed in a community for the duration of the epidemic (LaTour and Eichenwald Maki 2010, 442–443).

94. **c** Healthcare performance improvement philosophies most often focus on measuring performance in systems, processes, and outcomes. The foundations of caregiving, buildings, equipment, professional staff, and policies are all examples of systems (Shaw and Elliott 2012, 14).

95. **b** Healthcare performance improvement philosophies most often focus on measuring performance in systems, processes, and outcomes. The interrelated activities in healthcare organizations that promote effective and safe patient outcomes are examples of processes (Shaw and Elliott 2012, 14).

96. **a** Healthcare performance improvement philosophies most often focus on measuring performance in systems, processes, and outcomes. The results of care, treatment, and services are examples of outcomes (Shaw and Elliott 2012, 14).

97. **c** Performance measurement gives healthcare providers an indication of an organization's performance in relation to a specified process or outcome. A process measure has a scientific basis for it (Shaw and Elliott 2012, 16).

98. **a** An outcome measure may be the effect of care, treatment, or services on a customer (Shaw and Elliott 2012, 16).

99. **c** A process measure has a scientific basis for it. In this example, the percentage of antibiotics administered before surgery has been proven through evidence-based medicine so it is scientifically based (Shaw and Elliott 2012, 16).

100. **a** A check sheet is used to gather data on sample observations in order to detect patterns. When preparing to collect data, a team should consider the four W questions: Who will collect the data? What data will be collected? Where will the data be collected? When will the data be collected? Check sheets make it possible to systematically collect a large volume of data (Shaw and Elliott 2012, 47–48).

101. **a** Gender can be subdivided into two groups, male or female, or groups 1 or 2. This is an example of nominal or categorical data (Shaw and Elliott 2012, 48).

102. **b** Most survey data use a Lickert scale to quantify or rank statements. This is an example of the ordinal data (Shaw and Elliott 2012, 48).

103. **c** Examples of discrete data that must be represented by whole numbers include the number of children in a family or the number of unbillable patient accounts (Shaw and Elliott 2012, 48).

104. **d** Examples of continuous data include weight, blood pressure, and temperature. Continuous data are displayed on histograms (Shaw and Elliott 2012, 49).

105. **a** A survey is a common tool used in performance improvement to assess the level of satisfaction with a process by its customers. When designing a survey, the PI team must define the goal of the survey in clear and precise terms (Shaw and Elliott 2012, 98–100).

106. **b** An unstructured interview is not preplanned and flows with the conversation. This type of interview is helpful when the interviewer is trying to uncover preliminary problems that may need in-depth analysis and investigation (Shaw and Elliott 2012, 101).

107. **a** When using a structured interview you know exactly what questions to ask and understand the purpose and goal of each question so that a meaningful response can be recognized (Shaw and Elliott 2012, 101).

108. **c** Control charts can be used to measure key processes over time. Using a control chart focuses attention on any variation in the process (Shaw and Elliott 2012 62–63).

109. **c** Case managers review the condition of the patient to identify each patient's care needs and integrate patient data with the patient's course of treatment (Shaw and Elliott 2012, 112).

110. **a** Preadmission care planning is initiated when the patient's physician contacts a healthcare organization to schedule an episode of care service. The case manager reviews the patient's projected needs with the physician. Admission criteria are established based on a suggested diagnosis. The manager also may contact the patient directly to obtain further information (Shaw and Elliott 2012, 113).

111. **b** Photographic, chest x-ray film are all diagnostic image data that are based on analog, photographic films (LaTour and Eichenwald Maki 2010, 52).

112. **b** Text mining and data mining are the terms commonly used to describe the process of extracting and then quantifying and filtering free-text data and discrete data, respectively (LaTour and Eichenwald Maki 2010, 54).

113. **d** Providing the best care in the most effective manner and for the least cost is something every healthcare organization strives to do, and the patient wants the best outcome possible, which may be curative or not when they seek care. This is why the primary objective of quality in healthcare for both the patient and provider is to arrive at the desired outcome (Shaw and Elliott 2012, 108–109).

114. **b** The experts of managing the change process (for example, Deming, Juran, and Crosby) have developed methods to measure and monitor systems and processes in organizations. Their theories give managers methods to use in bringing about measured, focused change before crisis occurs. These methods were developed first in the business industry, and healthcare has struggled to adopt them (LaTour and Eichenwald Maki 2010, 518).

115. **b** Clinical performance is often measured around diagnosis, medical condition, or care processes along with outcomes. The relationship between the way care is provided and the outcomes or results of the medical intervention is the focus of clinical quality management (LaTour and Eichenwald Maki 2010, 518).

116. **c** The material safety data sheets (MSDSs) give detailed information about a material, including any hazards associated with the material. MSDSs must be available immediately to employees at locations where hazardous materials are used (Shaw and Elliott 2012, 244–250).

117. **b** Healthcare organizations need to be very clear about which abbreviations are not acceptable to use when writing or communicating medication orders. The organization's policy should also define whether or when the diagnosis, condition, or indication for use is included on a medication order (Shaw and Elliott 2012, 214).

118. **b** Like any organization, the medical staff, as a self-governing entity, needs to have structure. The medical staff bylaws provide an organizational structure to ensure communication with the governing body and high-quality patient care. Committees are used to help most medical staffs function. This committee structure is used to make credentialing and clinical privilege decisions (Brodnik et al. 2012 463–464).

119. **c** Risk management is a program designed to reduce or prevent injuries and accidents and to minimize or prevent financial loss to the organization (Shaw and Elliott 2012, 186).

120. **b** Severity indexing is the process of identifying the level of resource consumption based on factors of clinical evidence. The more complications and comorbid conditions present, the sicker the patient and the higher the resource consumption. This method of trying to judge the level of illness is useful for reimbursement, utilization, and quality of care programs (LaTour and Eichenwald Maki 2010, 525).

121. **c** Performance measures are quantifiable indicators used over time to determine whether structure, process, or outcome supports quality performance. They usually represent important aspects of care provided by the organization, department, or unit of service. Performance measure development has been a linchpin for clinical quality improvement (LaTour and Eichenwald Maki 2010, 532).

122. **a** The scope of performance measurement activities requires clarity. The important areas of service are usually based on volume, risk, or known problem. The population targeted must be clearly identified and defined, and the sample size must be representative and allow for valid and reliable statistical measurement. Descriptions of the raw data and data sources must be identified precisely so that everyone understands what the data elements will tell them. The medical record remains as the main data source (LaTour and Eichenwald Maki 2010, 552).

123. **b** Key to the implementation of an effective PI program is a written plan that systematically describes the structure and approach the organization will follow in the continuous assessment and improvement of its important systems, processes, and outcomes of care. Items commonly found in a plan include statement of mission and vision, objectives, values, leadership, organizational structure, methodologies, performance measures, communication, and annual plan appraisal (Shaw and Elliott 2012, 400).

124. **c** AHRQ began to develop outcome measures and was a resource in outcomes assessment. This agency has worked diligently to provide clinical evidence for best practice. In 2003, the AHRQ, together with Stanford-UCSF (University of California, San Francisco) Evidence-based Practice Center, developed a plan to analyze literature on QI strategies. These analyses focused on translating research into practice, concentrating on what would increase the rate of effective practices as applied to patient care in actual practice settings. The aim of this program is to close the quality gap (LaTour and Eichenwald Maki 2010, 523).

125. **b** The governing body is ultimately responsible for the quality of care provided in any organization. Today, governing bodies are more involved in QI efforts than ever before. Board members are seeking training, asking questions, and insisting on seeing data confirming that care is improving within their organization. When a board expresses interest and concern about the quality of care being provided, it sets the bar for medical staff, administrative, and staff involvement (Shaw and Elliott 2012, 318).

126. **c** Individuals involved in QI processes in healthcare organizations must determine who the customers are, what they want, and what must be done to meet their expectations. Expectations must translate into performance requirements so that healthcare professionals can evaluate whether customers' needs are being met. This leads to developing statements of expectation or performance called performance measures (Shaw and Elliott 2012, 84–85).

127. **c** Core performance measures are considered tools—standardized metrics—that provide an indication of an organization's performance. Core measures are defined as standardized sets of valid, reliable, and evidenced-based measures implemented by the Joint Commission (LaTour and Eichenwald Maki 2010, 537).

128. **b** The medical staff must lead the way in improving clinical and nonclinical processes used in organizations. Involvement of the medical staff in patient care review is critical. This means the medical staff is involved in measuring, assessing, and improving processes that depend on licensed physicians or other practitioners credentialed and privileged through the medical staff process. The use of blood and blood components, medication use, and surgical case are examples of these clinical QI activities (LaTour and Eichenwald Maki 2010, 544–545).

129. **c** Utilization management (sometimes referred to as case management) is a formal review of patient resource use. Data collected during this formal review help determine the appropriateness of the services provided. UM ensures the medical necessity of treatment provided and the cost-effective use of resources and identifies overuse or underuse of available services. Preadmission review, discharge planning, and retrospective review are all basic functions of the utilization management process. Claims management, review of potentially compensable events, and loss prevention are not basic functions of the utilization management process (Shaw and Elliott 2012, 112–115).

130. **b** Avidas Donabedian's QA model has been used and accepted for many years. The model's approach to the assessment of healthcare is based on the following three measures: Structure measures examine the organization's capability to provide services. Process measures look at how care or service is provided to patients. The activities or protocols of care have some impact on the patient's outcome. Outcome measures assess the end results of the care or services provided (LaTour and Eichenwald Maki 2010, 536–537).

131. **a** The medical staff and the healthcare organization should work together to provide an environment that reduces the risk of infections in both patients and healthcare providers. The healthcare organization should support activities that look for, prevent, and control infections. An infection review is done with the involvement of the medical staff. Information is collected regularly on endemic and epidemic healthcare-associated infections. As appropriate, the healthcare organization must report significant information to both internal groups and public health agencies (Shaw and Elliott 2012, 160–165).

132. **d** Risk management is a program designed to reduce or prevent injuries and accidents and to minimize or prevent financial loss to the organization (Shaw and Elliott 2012, 186).

133. **b** Clinical quality management involves the evaluation of direct patient care. Clinical performance is often measured around diagnosis, medical condition, or care processes along with outcomes. The relationship between the way care is provided and the outcomes or results of the medical intervention is the focus of clinical quality management (LaTour and Eichenwald Maki 2010, 518).

134. **c** A utilization management program helps ensure that patients receive appropriate care in an efficient and cost-effective manner (Casto and Layman 2011, 99–100).

135. **c** Discharge planning ensures that a patient is ready for placement in a nonacute setting when he or she leaves the facility. This process often begins either at preadmission or upon admission to ensure that the patient is placed or receives services needed at the time of discharge (Shaw and Elliott 2012, 113–115).

136. **a** The admission review is done at the time the patient is admitted to the facility. This review is done to determine or verify the medical necessity and appropriateness of admission (Shaw and Elliott 2012, 113).

137. **d** The preadmission review is done prior to the patient's admission. It is required by most managed care plans. Its purpose is to determine if the admission and procedure are medically necessary and appropriate in an acute care setting. The preadmission review identifies patients who are unsuitable for admission or for a particular procedure and then directs them to the appropriate care setting to obtain healthcare services (Shaw and Elliott 2012, 113).

138. **b** Continued-stay or concurrent review ensures that the patient is remaining in the facility because of medical necessity and is being treated appropriately. The review ensures that the patient is evaluated at preset intervals to determine the appropriateness of care rendered and that beds are utilized efficiently. The specific interval is commonly tied to the diagnosis and procedure (Shaw and Elliott 2012, 113).

139. **d** Many healthcare statistics are reported in the form of a ratio, proportion, or rate. These measures are used to report morbidity (illness), mortality (death), and natality (birthrate) at the local, state, and national levels (LaTour and Eichenwald Maki 2010, 424–425).

140. **b** Quantity standards (also called productivity standards) and quality standards (also known as service standards) are generally used by managers to monitor individual employee performance and the performance of a functional unit or the department as a whole. To properly communicate performance standards, managers need to make the distinction between quantitative and qualitative standards and identify examples of each for the HIS functions (LaTour and Eichenwald Maki 2010, 690).

141. **b** Quantity standards (also called productivity standards) and quality standards (also known as service standards) are generally used by managers to monitor individual employee performance and the performance of a functional unit or the department as a whole. To properly communicate performance standards, managers need to make the distinction between quantitative and qualitative standards and identify examples of each for the HIS functions (LaTour and Eichenwald Maki 2010, 690).

142. **d** Disease registries are collections of secondary data related to patients with a specific diagnosis, condition, or procedure. Registries are different from indexes in that they contain more extensive data. Index reports can usually be produced using data from the facility's existing databases. Registries often require more extensive data from the patient record. Each registry must define the cases that are to be included in it. This process is called case definition. In a trauma registry, for example, the case definition might be all patients admitted with a diagnosis falling into ICD-9-CM code numbers 800–959, the trauma diagnosis codes (LaTour and Eichenwald Maki 2010, 331).

143. **c** A proportion is a particular type of ratio in which x is a portion of the whole $(x + y)$. In a proportion, the numerator is always included in the denominator (LaTour and Eichenwald Maki 2010, 424–425).

144. **a** The Institutional Review Board (IRB) is a committee established to protect the rights and welfare of human research subjects involved in research activities. The IRB determines whether research that is conducted is appropriate and protects human subjects as they participate in this research. The primary focus of the IRB is not on whether the type of research is appropriate for the organization to conduct but upon whether or not human subjects are adequately protected (LaTour and Eichenwald Maki 2010, 492).

145. **d** A skewed distribution is asymmetrical. Skewness is the horizontal stretching of a frequency distribution to one side or the other so that one tail is longer than the other. The longer tail has more observations. Because the mean is sensitive to extreme observations, it moves in the direction of the long tail when a distribution is skewed. When the direction of the tail is off to the right, the distribution is positively skewed, or skewed to the right. When the direction of the tail is off to the left, the distribution is negatively skewed, or skewed to the left (LaTour and Eichenwald Maki 2010, 457–458).

146. **d** The range is the simplest measure of spread. It is the difference between the smallest and largest values in a frequency distribution:

$$\text{Range} = X_{\text{max}} - X_{\text{min}}$$

For this scenario, the range is 1 to 29 (29 – 1) or 28 (LaTour and Eichenwald Maki 2010, 456–457).

147. **c** The median is the midpoint of a frequency distribution and falls in the ordinal scale of measurement. It is the point at which 50 percent of the observations fall above and 50 percent fall below. If an odd number of observations is in the frequency distribution, the median is the middle number. In this data set, 8 is the middle number (LaTour and Eichenwald Maki 2010, 455–456).

148. **c** The median offers the following three advantages: relatively easy to calculate; based on the whole distribution and not just a portion of it, as is the case with the mode; and unlike the mean, it is not influenced by extreme values or unusual outliers in the frequency distribution (LaTour and Eichenwald Maki 2010, 456).

149. **a** The discrepancy is between the researcher's use of the term "anonymous" in the informed consent and the researcher's intent to track respondents. Anonymity demands that the researcher cannot link the response and the responder. The code would link the respondents to their data, so their data would no longer be anonymous (LaTour and Eichenwald Maki 2010, 507).

150. **d** The proportionate mortality ratio (PMR) is a measure of mortality due to a specific cause for a specific time period. In the formula for calculating the PMR, the numerator is the number of deaths due to a specific disease for a specific time period, and the denominator is the number of deaths from all causes for the same time period. The proportionate mortality ratio for diabetes mellitus = $73,249 / 2,443,387 = 0.03$ (LaTour and Eichenwald Maki 2010, 441).

151. **c** A skewed distribution is asymmetrical. Skewness is the horizontal stretching of a frequency distribution to one side or the other so that one tail is longer than the other. The longer tail has more observations. Because the mean is sensitive to extreme observations, it moves in the direction of the long tail when a distribution is skewed. When the direction of the tail is off to the right, the distribution is positively skewed, or skewed to the right. When the direction of the tail is off to the left, the distribution is negatively skewed, or skewed to the left (LaTour and Eichenwald Maki 2010, 457–458).

152. **d** Respect for persons requires that individuals be treated as autonomous human beings and not used as a means to an end. Elements of autonomy include the ability to understand and process information and the freedom to volunteer for research without coercion or undue influence from others. Respect for persons requires informed consent and respecting the privacy of research subjects (LaTour and Eichenwald Maki 2010, 563).

153. **c** The standard deviation is the most widely used measure of variability in descriptive statistics. The standard deviation is easy to interpret and is the most preferred measure of dispersion for frequency distributions (LaTour and Eichenwald Maki 2010, 457).

154. **a** External users of patient data are individuals and institutions outside the facility. Examples include state data banks and federal agencies. States have laws that mandate cases of patients with diseases such as tuberculosis and AIDS be reported to the state department of health. Moreover, the federal government collects data from the states on vital events such as births and deaths (LaTour and Eichenwald Maki 2010, 330).

155. **a** Bar charts are used to display data from one or more variables. The bars may be drawn vertically or horizontally. Bar charts are used for nominal or ordinal variables. In this case, you would be displaying the average length of stay by service and then within each service have a bar for each gender (LaTour and Eichenwald Maki 2010, 446).

156. **b** The structure of the database must be designed carefully. In a well-designed database, data is entered once and stored in one place. Anyone who accesses the data gets the most updated version. A poorly designed database can lead to redundant data and information errors, which in turn can lead to poor management or patient care decisions (LaTour and Eichenwald Maki 2010, 125).

157. **d** Quality has several components, including the following: appropriateness, the right care is provided at the right time; technical excellence, the right care is provided in the right manner; accessibility, the right care can be obtained when it is needed; and acceptability, the patients are satisfied (LaTour and Eichenwald Maki 2010, 33–34).

158. **c** Hospital-acquired (nosocomial) infection rates may be calculated for the entire hospital or for a specific unit in the hospital. They also may be calculated for the specific types of infections. Ideally, the hospital should strive for an infection rate of 0.0 percent. The formula for calculating the hospital-acquired, or nosocomial, infection rate is: Total number of hospital-acquired infections for a given period / Total number of discharges, including deaths, for the same period × 100 (LaTour and Eichenwald Maki 2010, 434).

159. **a** A disease index is a listing in diagnosis code number order for patients discharged from the facility during a particular time period. Each patient's diagnoses are converted from a verbal description to a numerical code, usually using a coding system such as the ICD-9-CM (LaTour and Eichenwald Maki 2010, 331).

160. **c** The nosocomial infection rate is (4 × 100) / 57 = 400 / 57 = 7.0% Hospital-acquired (nosocomial) infection rates may be calculated for the entire hospital. They also may be calculated for the specific types of infections. Ideally, the hospital should strive for an infection rate of 0.0 percent (LaTour and Eichenwald Maki 2010, 434).

161. **c** The popularity of these quality improvement approaches has demonstrated the growing importance of customer satisfaction (LaTour and Eichenwald Maki 2010, 628).

162. **c** Most states require the reporting of unusual events or other public health prevention and control programs. Any unusual event, unexpected occurrence, or accident resulting in death or life-threatening or serious injury to the patient that is not related to a natural course of the patient's illness or underlying condition is usually reported (Brodnik et al. 2012, 282).

163. **d** Epidemiological data is used to describe health-related issues or events such as disease trends found in specific populations or general analytics of population health (LaTour and Eichenwald Maki 2010, 89).

164. **d** The nominal group technique gives each member of the team the opportunity to select which ideas identified from the affinity diagram process are the most important. This technique allows groups to narrow the focus of discussion or make decisions without getting involved in extended, circular discussions during which more vocal members dominate (Shaw and Elliott 2012, 20–21).

165. **b** The Pareto chart is based on the Pareto Principle, which states that 20 percent of the sources of the problem are responsible for 80 percent of the actual problems. By concentrating on the vital few sources, a large number of actual problems can be eliminated (LaTour and Eichenwald Maki 2010, 705).

166. **a** Clinical data are the most common type of health information and document the signs, symptoms, diagnoses, impressions, treatments, and outcomes of the care process. They are captured during diagnosis and treatment and stored in the medical record. Clinical data serve a variety of industry needs beyond direct patient care, including reimbursement, planning, and research (Odom-Wesley et al. 2009, 92, 98).

167. **b** A histogram is used to display a frequency distribution. It is different from a bar graph in that a bar graph is used to display data that fall into groups or categories (nominal or ordinal data) when the categories are noncontinuous or discrete (LaTour and Eichenwald Maki 2010, 448).

168. **a** Clinical information systems (or applications) contain primarily clinical or health-related data that are used to diagnose, treat, monitor, and manage patient care. Examples of clinical applications include ancillary departmental systems (such as pharmacy, radiology, and laboratory medicine) as well as EMR systems, CPOE, medication administration, and nursing documentation (LaTour and Eichenwald Maki 2010, 144).

169. **a** Healthcare organizations are under increased pressure to control costs and improve efficiency. At the same time, they are experiencing increased demands to ensure patient safety, reduce medical errors, improve the quality of care, promote access, and ensure compliance with privacy and security regulations. Many healthcare organizations are looking to information system (IS) technology to help them respond to these pressures and provide high-quality services in a more cost-effective manner (LaTour and Eichenwald Maki 2010, 144).

170. **d** The three primary barriers are the high cost of acquiring and supporting systems, a lack of sufficient standards and interoperability concerns, and organizational and behavioral resistance (LaTour and Eichenwald Maki 2010, 145).

171. **b** It is critical that the organization's IS plans be well aligned and integrated with its overall organizational strategic plans. To develop a blueprint for IS technology, the healthcare organization should engage in strategic IS planning (LaTour and Eichenwald Maki 2010, 145).

172. **c** The CIO is responsible for helping to lead the strategic IS planning process, managing the major functional units within the IS department, and overseeing the management of information resources throughout the enterprise (LaTour and Eichenwald Maki 2010, 153).

173. **d** An environmental assessment should be performed to explore emerging technologies and their potential impact on the ways the healthcare organization delivers its services. This assessment should include both the external and internal environment (LaTour and Eichenwald Maki 2010, 146).

174. **c** A well-constructed RFP serves two important purposes. One is to solidify the planning information and organizational requirements into a single document and the other is to provide valuable insights into the vendor's operations and products and to level the playing field in terms of asking all the vendors the same questions. This process requires skill and time (Amatayakul 2012, 385).

175. **c** During the implementation phase of the SDLC, a comprehensive plan for implementing the new system is developed. This plan would include all plans for training managers, technical staff, and other end-users (LaTour and Eichenwald Maki 2010, 150–151).

176. **a** During the analysis phase, the need for a new information system is explored further, problems with the existing system are solidified, and user needs are identified (LaTour and Eichenwald Maki 2010, 149).

177. **b** During the implementation phase of the SDLC, a comprehensive plan for implementing the new system is developed. This plan would include all plans for training managers, technical staff, and other end-users (LaTour and Eichenwald Maki 2010, 150–151).

178. **a** Throughout the implementation process, many tasks or activities may occur simultaneously; others will need to be completed before other activities can begin. Because of the number of different tasks occurring, it is generally a good idea for the project manager to use a Gantt chart or project management software that identifies the major tasks, their estimated start and completion dates, the individuals responsible for performing them, and the resources needed to complete them (LaTour and Eichenwald Maki 2010, 151).

179. **d** The CIO is responsible for helping to lead the strategic IS planning process, managing the major functional units within the IS department, and overseeing the management of information resources throughout the enterprise (LaTour and Eichenwald Maki 2010, 153).

180. **a** Best-of-breed is when an organization has acquired the "best" products from various vendors. The result is that each individual organization unit may be happy with its chosen product, but as the organization moves toward adding clinical components that rely on the various other systems as a source of data or to which data must be sent, the challenge to exchange such data can be overwhelming (Amatayakul 2012, 375–376).

181. **b** The Federated–consistent database model is essentially the same as the consolidated model of data being stored in separate data vaults, yet is it still managed centrally (Amatayakul 2012, 592–593).

182. **c** For whatever architecture an HIE organization may have, there needs to be a way to identify participants, which may include individual providers, representatives of payer organizations, and patients/consumers, as well as organizational entities and their information systems. This service is called registry and directory (Amatayakul 2012, 594).

183. **b** The opposite of best-of-breed is best-of-fit. In this situation, virtually (though not absolutely) all applications are provided by a single vendor. This frequently makes it easier to add new applications from that vendor, but potentially even more difficult to add products from other vendors. Many organizations find their best-of-fit financial/administrative and operational system vendor is not as strong in EHR as they would desire. Alternatively, best-of-breed organizations find it difficult and costly to sustain this approach (Amatayakul 2012, 178).

184. **a** Free text is the entry of narrative data, primarily via keyboarding, although dictation, voice recognition, and handwriting recognition are possible. Dictation uses a third party to transcribe the data, so there will always be a delay factor in seeing the results (Amatayakul 2012, 320–321).

185. **b** Because there is no mandated unique patient identifier, ensuring that the HIE organization can identify the right patient as it seeks to exchange information is a process of identity matching (Amatayakul 2012, 594).

186. **a** Implementation of an EHR component, or functions of a component, in one or a few organizational units at a time with a plan to follow on with full roll-out in the same manner is called a phased roll-out (Amatayakul 2012, 405).

187. **a** Parallel processing is a turnover strategy where the organization continues processing in manual form as well as electronic form. The intent is to validate the electronic processing against the manual processing (Amatayakul 2012, 405).

188. **d** Straight turnover refers to having everyone in the designated group go live at one time, with paper processes ceasing virtually immediately after go-live. This is the most typical form of turnover for EHRs because most organizations find that any reliance on former paper processing not only ends up being too time-consuming but also sends a message that the system is not to be trusted (Amatayakul 2012, 407).

189. **b** The implementation of all aspects of the EHR component (or entire EHR in an ambulatory setting) in all organizational units virtually simultaneously (Amatayakul 2012, 405).

190. **b** Because of the number of tasks and their complexity and dependencies in EHR implementation, it is important to have an issues management program. An issues management program serves to receive and document issues and track them to their resolution (Amatayakul 2012, 411).

191. **c** Within healthcare, standard protocols that support communication between nonintegrated applications are often referred to as messaging standards, also called interoperability standards or data exchange standards. Messaging standards provide the tools to map proprietary formats to one another and more easily accomplish the exchange of data (Amatayakul 2012, 310).

192. **c** Report generation consists of the formatting and/or structuring of captured information. It is the process of analyzing, organizing, and presenting recorded patient information for authentication and inclusion in the patient's healthcare record (LaTour and Eichenwald Maki 2010, 117).

193. **c** HL7 adopted the term "EHR" in its EHR-System Functional Model and has described a highly functional system. EHR is the only term used by the federal government in its efforts to promote adoption of HIT, including requiring "interoperable EHRs" (Amatayakul 2012, 226–227).

194. **a** Message format standards ensure that the structure and format of data are the same, as they are being transmitted from one system to another. This data structure and format is called syntax. Each proprietary system has its own syntax. For systems to exchange data or "talk" to one another, the syntax must be made the same (LaTour and Eichenwald Maki 2010, 243).

195. **b** In a transactional system, the database has been constructed according to well-established principles of relational database design, in particular, normalization. Normalization seeks to eliminate redundancy in data storage (Amatayakul 2012, 274).

196. **a** When developing the data elements that go into a database, the fields should be normalized. Normalization is breaking the data elements into the level of detail desired by the facility. For example, last name and first name should be in separate fields as should city, state, and zip code (Sayles and Trawick 2010, 91).

197. **d** A clinical data repository is a database that has been developed using a consistent clinical data model and clinical vocabulary and provides accurate clinical data from the various patient care systems. The clinical repository requires that the other health information and patient care systems be integrated with it to allow data to flow between it and the other systems. Thus, the clinical repository is like the data warehouse in that it serves as a database for storing data from transactional systems (LaTour and Eichenwald Maki 2010, 608).

198. **c** The MPI functions as the primary guide to locating pertinent demographic data about the patient and his or her health record number. Without the information contained in the MPI, it would be almost impossible to locate a patient's health record in most organizations that use a numeric filing system. The MPI is the permanent record of every patient ever seen in the healthcare entity. The amount of information contained on each patient in the MPI varies from facility to facility. However, the basic information usually includes patient's last, first, and middle names; patient's health record number(s); patient's date of birth; patient's gender; and dates of encounter. Additional information such as address, telephone number, and attending physician for each encounter also may be recorded (Odom-Wesley et al. 2009, 78–79).

199. **c** Data mining is the process of probing and extracting business data and information from a data warehouse and then quantifying and filtering the data for analysis purposes (LaTour and Eichenwald Maki 2010, 66).

200. **a** A local area network (LAN) is a group of computers typically connected within a relatively small geographic area, such as an office, building, or campus. Connectivity is generally achieved through dedicated cable (Amatayakul 2012, 298).

201. **b** A group of computers that connect across great geographical distances, often using telephone or cable services for connectivity is a wide area network (WAN) (Amatayakul 2012, 298).

202. **c** A wireless local area network (WLAN) is a group of wireless devices that connect to a LAN via radio waves (Amatayakul 2012, 298).

203. **a** There are two types of topology: physical and logical. A physical topology is the way in which network devices are connected. Networks are generally arranged in one of three topologies: bus topology, star topology, and ring topology. Logical topology describes how data are transmitted through the physical devices (Amatayakul 2012, 300).

204. **b** An ethernet is a family of frame-based computer networking technologies that currently are the most widely used topologies for LANs (Amatayakul 2012, 300).

205. **d** Trunk lines (T-lines) are the backbone of long-distance, packet-switched network transmission that transmit data in digital form. They come in a variety of speeds and may also carry voice (Amatayakul 2012, 302).

206. **b** Infrared light (for example, Bluetooth) is used to carry information between devices in a network. It is popularly used between PDAs and cell phones to "beam" data from one device to another, and in healthcare between medical devices and information systems (Amatayakul 2012, 301).

207. **c** Bus topology is the simplest network topology, connecting one device to another along a "backbone" (Amatayakul 2012, 300).

208. **a** Star topology is one physical topology of a network and uses a central hub as a traffic cop (Amatayakul 2012, 300).

209. **d** Input/output devices are considered peripheral devices because they are separate from the central processing unit of the computer, even if they are housed in the single casing like a notebook computer. Examples of input devices are keyboards, mouse, touch pad, light pen, optical character recognition, etc. (Amatayakul 2012, 288–289).

210. **d** Portable devices require a battery for their power, which is perhaps one of their main drawbacks for use in a 24/7 environment, or even in an 8-hour day. Most portable computers do not have sufficient battery power to last 8 hours (Amatayakul 2012, 289–290).

211. **b** Secondary storage may be available continuously (online) to the CPU for real-time access to data or physically separated (offline) and require online loading to be connected to the CPU. The term drive is often used to describe the device that runs a secondary storage medium (Amatayakul 2012, 291–292).

212. **c** One configuration that is commonly used is called *redundant arrays of inexpensive (or independent) disks* (RAID). RAID comes in different levels; although the names of the levels are not standardized, there are typically from two to five levels (Amatayakul 2012, 292–293).

213. **b** Mainframe computers use a single large computer with many terminals directly connected to it and sharing the resources of the single computer (Amatayakul 2012, 295).

214. **a** Client/server architecture is the predominant form of computer architecture used in healthcare associations today. In client/server architecture, certain computers (servers) have been configured to perform most of the processing and resource-intensive tasks, while other computers (clients), which generally are less-powerful computers, capture, view, and perform limited processes on data (Amatayakul 2012, 296).

215. **b** Web-based, or web service architecture (WSA), uses the technology concepts of the Internet and World Wide Web for local area (intranets) or wide area (extranet) network design (Amatayakul 2012, 297).

216. **c** *Web browser-based* or *web native systems* are systems where companies have either written or rewritten their systems' code using HTML, SGML, XML, or Java and its derivatives (LaTour and Eichenwald Maki 2010, 61).

217. **c** Online analytical processing (OLAP) is an application architecture that was developed to explore the multidimensional aspects of such business data. OLAP stores the data in a multidimensional data structure and enables the user to examine and view the data along dimensions that may be specific to the context and will be defined by the business rules of the organization (LaTour and Eichenwald Maki 2010, 609–610).

218. **b** Data mining is the process of probing and extracting business data and information from a data warehouse and then quantifying and filtering the data for analysis purposes (LaTour and Eichenwald Maki 2010, 66).

219. **b** Linkage analysis portrays relationships discovered within data sets by a linked network graph. Many healthcare organizations as well as government agencies are investigating linkage analysis as a DSS tool for containing the increasing cost of healthcare due to fraud and abuse (LaTour and Eichenwald Maki 2010, 607).

220. **b** Data mining is the process of sorting through the organization's data to identify unusual patterns or to apply analytical models that will assist in predicting future events. Current applications of data-mining activities in healthcare include models to support fraud detection, utilization review, and clinical pathways (LaTour and Eichenwald Maki 2010, 600).

221. **b** To enhance retrieval of scanned documents, some form of indexing needs to take place in order to organize the documents for easy retrieval. Ideally, each form that is scanned or otherwise created should have a bar code or some other forms recognition feature, or features, associated with it (Amatayakul 2012, 444).

222. **c** A picture archiving and communication system (PACS) is used to store radiology and other clinical images (Amatayakul 2012, 165).

223. **a** Unit numbering storage is a health record identification system in which the patient receives a unique medical record number at the time of the first encounter that is used for all subsequent encounters (LaTour and Eichenwald Maki 2010, 218).

224. **d** A terminal-digit filing system is a health record identification and filing system in which the last digit or group of digits (terminal digits) in the health record number determines file placement (LaTour and Eichenwald Maki 2010, 218–219).

225. **a** One benefit of the unit filing system is that all records for a specific patient, both inpatient and outpatient, are filed together (LaTour and Eichenwald Maki 2010, 218–219).

226. **a** The microfilm jacket has the advantage of serving as an individual folder for storing the records of one patient. Additional filmed images can be added to the jacket or changed. The jackets are usually 4 × 6 inches and have a strip at the top on which to record the patient's name and number (LaTour and Eichenwald Maki 2010, 223).

227. **a** If an EHR is to provide clinical decision support it requires two things: structured data and a clinical data repository (LaTour and Eichenwald Maki 2010, 233).

228. **a** The continuity of care record (CCR) helps standardize clinical content for sharing between providers. A CCR allows documentation of care delivery from one healthcare experience to another (LaTour and Eichenwald Maki 2010, 179).

229. **c**   The capability to retrieve documents from an electronic document management system (EDMS) is determined by the underlying technology used to store the documents. In addition to bar codes on medical record documents, optical character recognition (OCR) may be available to enhance the accuracy of indexing features on forms (Amatayakul 2012, 443–444).

230. **b**   Case finding includes the methods used to identify the patients who have been seen and treated in the facility for the particular disease or condition of interest to the registry. After cases have been identified, extensive information is abstracted from the paper-based patient record into the registry database or fed from other databases and entered into the registry database (LaTour and Eichenwald Maki 2010, 331).

231. **b**   The National Ambulatory Medical Care Survey includes data collected by a sample of office-based physicians and their staffs from the records of patients seen in a one-week reporting period. Data included are demographic data, the patient's reason for visit, the diagnoses, diagnostic and screening services, therapeutic and preventive services, ambulatory surgical procedures, and medications and injections, in addition to information on the visit disposition and time spent with the physician (LaTour and Eichenwald Maki 2010, 339).

232. **d**   Interface is the hardware, software, data definitions, and standard messaging protocols required for data to be exchanged among separate computer systems. In this case, the interface allows the information to pass from the R-ADT system to the laboratory vendor system (Amatayakul 2012, 308).

233. **b**   SQL includes both Data Dictionary Language and Data Manipulation Language components and is used to create and manipulate relational databases (Sayles and Trawick 2010, 177–178).

234. **c**   Firewalls are hardware and software security devices situated between the routers of a private and public network. They are designed to protect computer networks from unauthorized outsiders (LaTour and Eichenwald Maki 2010, 79).

235. **a**   An object-oriented database is derived from object-oriented programming and has no single inherent structure. The structure for any given class or type of object can be anything a programmer finds useful—a linked list, a set, an array, etc. An object may contain different degrees of complexity, making use of multiple types and multiple structures (Amatayakul 2012, 267).

236. **d**   Managing data storage has become an increasingly important issue. Where in the past data were retained online for, at most, a matter of days after discharge or a visit, and a backup was made daily and stored on tape, an EHR virtually demands that data be retained online forever, be instantaneously retrievable, and be backed up continuously—both locally and in a remote environment for disaster recovery (LaTour and Eichenwald Maki 2010, 249).

237. **a**   Databases contain rules known as integrity constraints that must be satisfied by the stored data. Data integrity happens when all of the data in the database conform to all integrity constraint rules. These constraints help ensure that the originally entered data and changes to these data follow certain rules. After the parameters for the types of integrity have been set within the database, users cannot violate them (LaTour and Eichenwald Maki 2010, 134).

238. **c**   User access control features within the database are designed to limit access to the database or some portion of it. Assigning access privileges can be done according to user groups or on an individual basis. The highest level of privilege is the administrative level, which should be reserved for the database administrator. Persons with administrative permissions can change the underlying structure of the database (LaTour and Eichenwald Maki 2010, 134).

239. **d** Firewalls are hardware and software security devices situated between the routers of a private and public network. They are designed to protect computer networks from unauthorized outsiders. However, they also can be used to protect entities within a single network, for example, to block laboratory technicians from getting into payroll records. Without firewalls, IT departments would have to deploy multiple-enterprise security programs that would soon become difficult to manage and maintain (LaTour and Eichenwald Maki 2010, 79).

240. **a** Validity refers to the accuracy of the data. (The extent to which data correspond to the actual state of affairs or that an instrument measures what it purports to measure.) (LaTour and Eichenwald Maki 2010, 342–343).

241. **b** The use of a password is a method to identify the author of the data. HIPAA Security Guidance offers recommendations for possible risk management strategies including two-factor identification, increased backup, and password protection for all files (LaTour and Eichenwald Maki 2010, 254).

242. **a** Access control is a critical function within HIM relative to information security. This function maps the relationship between information and the individuals authorized to use it. It may be established at a variety of levels (LaTour and Eichenwald Maki 2010, 91).

243. **b** Protecting the security and privacy of data in the database is called authorization management. Two of the important aspects of authorization management are user access control and usage monitoring (Rob and Coronel 2010; LaTour and Eichenwald Maki 2010, 134).

244. **c** Firewalls are hardware and software security devices situated between the routers of a private and public network. They are designed to protect computer networks from unauthorized outsiders. However, they also can be used to protect entities within a single network, for example, to block laboratory technicians from getting into payroll records. Without firewalls, IT departments would have to deploy multiple-enterprise security programs that would soon become difficult to manage and maintain (LaTour and Eichenwald Maki 2010, 79).

245. **b** E-health is the application of e-commerce to the healthcare industry. E-health offers businesses and consumers the opportunity to provide or engage in a number of services, including: PHRs; patient appointment scheduling; patient registration; pre-visit health screening, evaluations, and assessments; post-visit patient education; information on health conditions, diseases, wellness, or new healthcare developments; and support for handheld, point-of-care devices (LaTour and Eichenwald Maki 2010, 75).

246. **d** A web portal is a single point of personalized access (an entryway) through which to find and deliver information (content), applications, and services. Web portals began in the consumer market as an integration strategy rather than a solution. Portals offered users of the large, public, online Internet service provider websites, such as AOL, fast, centralized access (via a web browser) to an array of Internet services and information found on those websites (LaTour and Eichenwald Maki 2010, 61).

247. **c** EMPIs provide access to multiple repositories of information from overlapping patient populations that are maintained in separate systems and databases. This occurs through an indexing scheme to all unique patient identification numbers and information in all the organizations' databases. As such, EMPIs become the cornerstones of healthcare system integration projects (LaTour and Eichenwald Maki 2010, 57–58).

248. **d**   The clinician/physician web portals first were seen as a way for clinicians to easily access (via a web browser) the healthcare provider organizations' multiple sources of structured and unstructured data from any network-connected device. Like clinical workstations, clinician/physician web portals evolved into an effective medium for providing access to multiple applications as well as the data (LaTour and Eichenwald Maki 2010, 62).

249. **d**   Clinical/medical decision support systems are data driven. They assist clinicians in applying new information to patient care through the analysis of patient-specific clinical/medical variables. Clinical/medical decision support systems can be characterized by providing reminders and alerts, clinical guideline advice, therapy critiquing, or benchmarking tools (LaTour and Eichenwald Maki 2010, 67).

250. **a**   If an organization is adopting an EHR where there are considerable discrete data and a repository supporting CDS, it may want to abstract some or all of certain records so that the data are not only accessible for viewing, but also are available for processing (LaTour and Eichenwald Maki 2010, 266).

251. **a**   Healthcare organizations find it effective to mount a notebook computer to a cart and move it with the user. These sometimes are affectionately called computers on wheels (COWs) or wireless on wheels (WOWs) (LaTour and Eichenwald Maki 2010, 247).

252. **a**   This is one of many definitions of a decision support system. Because the goals involved in these systems have such breadth, no universally agreed-upon definition exists, but this is a good working definition and captures the important characteristics commonly identified for decision support systems (LaTour and Eichenwald Maki 2010, 600).

253. **d**   The inference engine is a module that can apply and link the appropriate rules together based on the inputs provided by the user (Amatayakul 2012, 484).

254. **c**   A data flow diagram is a diagram of how data flows in the database. The data flow diagram is a good way to show management and other nontechnical users the system design (Sayles and Trawick 2010, 97).

255. **a**   A benefits realization study is an evaluation of the benefits that have accrued from the EHR investment. It may be performed at specific milestones in the life of the project and used to help in future systems planning, designing, and implementing (Amatayakul 2012, 345).

256. **c**   A data repository is a database that is developed in an open format, thus allowing the facility to use it for multiple systems. The data repository is updated by the various systems in real time, thus providing users with access to the most current information available (Sayles and Trawick 2010, 100).

257. **d**   EDMS allows the ROI function to be shifted into decentralized areas including off-site clinics (Amatayakul 2012, 436).

258. **b**   A graphical user interface (GUI) is a style of computer interface in which typed commands are replaced by images that represent tasks. For example, this would allow the user to point, click, drag, and drop icon objects on the computer screen to accomplish desired tasks. Input devices include the standard keyboard and the computer mouse (Sayles and Trawick 2010, 12, 263).

259. **c**   A vocabulary standard is a common definition for medical terms to encourage consistent descriptions of an individual's condition in the health record (Sayles and Trawick 2010, 255).

260. **d** A data dictionary is a descriptive list of the data elements to be collected in an information system or database whose purpose is to ensure consistency of terminology (LaTour and Eichenwald Maki 2010, 131).

261. **a** Regional health information organizations (RHIOs) developed and maintained HIE standards in an attempt to share information and make it available where needed. These organizations bring together healthcare stakeholders within a defined region and govern the HIE process for the purpose of improving care in that community. As sophistication and utility of the Internet (based on standards) increases, there will be a number of new standards development activities emerging that affect health information management in all settings. The concept of a national health information infrastructure (NHII) is designed to bring information to and aid communication among all stakeholders in the process. The infrastructure requires technology investment for success but also requires fundamental change in business process, information sharing, and adoption of standards (LaTour and Eichenwald Maki 2010, 172).

262. **c** Brainstorming can be conducted in a structured or an unstructured way. This is an example of structured brainstorming. In unstructured brainstorming the members of the team offer ideas as they come to mind (Shaw and Elliott 2012, 20).

263. **c** The rectangle with double lines on the side in a flowchart is a predefined process icon. This symbol represents the formal procedure that participants are expected to carry out the same way every time (Shaw and Elliott 2012, 166–167).

264. **d** The symbol is called the manual input icon in flowcharting. This symbol represents points in the flowchart description of the process where the participants must record data in paper- or computer-based formats (Shaw and Elliott 2012, 167).

265. **c** Brainstorming can be conducted in a structured or an unstructured way. In structured brainstorming, the leader solicits input from team members by going from one to the next around the table or room. Each team member comments on the issue in turn or passes until the next round. This process continues until participants have no new ideas to suggest or until the time period set in the meeting's agenda has elapsed. In unstructured brainstorming, the members of the team offer ideas as they come to mind (Shaw and Elliott 2012, 20).

266. **a** Affinity diagrams are used to organize and prioritize ideas after the initial brainstorming session. This type of diagram is useful when the team generates a large amount of information. The team members agree on the primary categories or groupings from the brainstorming session, and then secondary ideas are listed under each primary category (Shaw and Elliott 2012, 20).

267. **b** The charge description master contains elements such as department and item number, item description, revenue code, HCPCS code, price, and activity status (Casto and Layman 2011, 251).

268. **d** Kinesthetic learners prefer to practice (LaTour and Eichenwald Maki 2010, 753).

269. **c** The CD-ROM/DVD-ROM constitutes about 48 percent of e-learning delivery methods, while web-based is 41 percent, and 11 percent is via computer or other means. Electronic training is most successful when there is a large audience to train, employees are geographically dispersed at several sites and/or work varied schedules, just-in-time training is required, and the purpose is to gain knowledge or learn applications (LaTour and Eichenwald Maki 2010, 756).

270. **c** Fayol's management functions have persisted with some variation into modern organizations and identify key functions that define the manager's role. These managerial functions were planning, organizing, leading, and controlling (LaTour and Eichenwald Maki 2010, 626).

271. **b** Each supervisor has a certain number of people who report to him or her, which is referred to as the span of management or the span of control (LaTour and Eichenwald Maki 2010, 630).

272. **b** Internal procedures include brainstorming, revisiting important decisions, monitoring the degree or consensus and disagreement, rotating the devil's advocate role, and actively seeking contradictory information. External procedures include discussing decisions with outside experts and nonteam members and inviting external observers to provide feedback on meetings, decisions, and team processes. Such procedures increase awareness of group processes and enhance skills at arriving at better decisions (LaTour and Eichenwald Maki 2010, 638).

273. **b** People are most receptive when feedback is solicited rather than imposed on them (LaTour and Eichenwald Maki 2010, 641).

274. **b** The basic systems model demonstrates that a system is made up of the components such as inputs and feedback. They are open systems because they are affected by what is going on around them and must adjust as the environment changes. These are not related to alternate work scheduling. Compressed workweek, telecommuting, and flextime are examples of alternate work scheduling (LaTour and Eichenwald Maki 2010, 686).

275. **a** A job procedure is a structured, action-oriented list of sequential steps involved in carrying out a specific job or solving a problem (LaTour and Eichenwald Maki 2010, 687).

276. **b** Effective management involves discerning what work is to be done, what performance standards are achievable and appropriate, how performance can be measured in terms of efficiency and effectiveness, and how performance can be monitored for variances from the standards set (LaTour and Eichenwald Maki 2010, 689).

277. **a** The next step in monitoring and measuring outcome performance is to compare current performance against established goals (standards) (LaTour and Eichenwald Maki 2010, 698).

278. **c** Qualitative standards specify the level of service quality expected from a function, such as accuracy rate. For example, assignment of diagnostic and procedure codes for inpatient records is at least 98 percent accurate (LaTour and Eichenwald Maki 2010, 690).

279. **c** There are several laws that affect discrimination in employment on the basis of race, color, religion, age, sex, national origin, citizenship status, and veterans status. Most organizations would like to hire someone whose vision for the organization is in line with their own vision (Brodnik et al. 2012, 476–477).

280. **b** The Americans with Disabilities Act of 1990 protects individuals with disabilities. Employees must be able to perform the necessary functions of a job with "reasonable accommodations," which include modifications to the workplace or conditions of employment so that a disabled worker can perform the job (Brodnik et al. 2012, 478).

281. **c** Collective bargaining is a process through which a contract is negotiated that sets forth the relationship between the employees and the healthcare organization. In a unionized facility, there will be a union steward who represents the employee in grievance and other similar situations (Brodnik et al. 2012, 483).

282. **d**   The Occupation Safety and Health Administration (OSHA) requires employers to create a safe working environment and comply with health standards for all employees (Brodnik et al. 2012, 484–485).

283. **b**   A balance sheet is a snapshot of the accounting equation at a point in time (LaTour and Eichenwald Maki 2010, 785–786).

284. **a**   An income statement summarizes the organization's revenue and expense transactions during the fiscal year. The income statement can be prepared at any point in time and reflects results up to that point. The income statement contains only income and expense accounts and reflects only the activity for the current fiscal year (LaTour and Eichenwald Maki 2010, 785).

285. **b**   Variances are often calculated on the monthly budget report. The organization's policies and procedures manual defines unacceptable variances or variances that must be explained. In identifying variances, it is important to recognize whether the variance is favorable or unfavorable and whether it is temporary or permanent (LaTour and Eichenwald Maki 2010, 799).

286. **b**   The capital budget looks at long-term investments. Such investments are usually related to improvements in the facility infrastructure, expansion of services, or replacement of existing assets. Capital investments focus on either the appropriateness of an investment (given the facility's investment guidelines) or choosing among different opportunities to invest. The capital budget is the facility's plan for allocating resources over and above the operating budget (LaTour and Eichenwald Maki 2010, 800).

287. **b**   Expenses are recorded in the same period as the associated revenue, thereby matching the expenses and revenues (LaTour and Eichenwald Maki 2010, 775).

288. **d**   An asset is something that is owned or due to be received. In a transaction, the compensation that has been earned by providing goods or services becomes an asset as soon as it has been earned. Examples of assets include cash, inventory, accounts receivable, buildings, and equipment (LaTour and Eichenwald Maki 2010, 779).

289. **b**   The purchase order system ensures that purchases have been properly authorized prior to ordering. Authorization is often tied to dollar limits or the budget process. Purchase orders are numbered sequentially so all orders can be verified (LaTour and Eichenwald Maki 2010, 782).

290. **d**   The Financial Accounting Standards Board (FASB) is an independent organization that sets accounting standards for businesses in the private sector. Its counterpart, the Government Accounting Standards Board (GASB), sets standards for accounting for government entities. The FASB promulgates the rules by which financial data are compiled, reported, reviewed, and audited. These rules, which include the conceptual framework, are referred to as generally accepted accounting principles (GAAP) and generally accepted auditing standards (GAAS) (LaTour and Eichenwald Maki 2010, 775).

291. **a**   The arithmetic difference between total revenue and total expenses is net income (LaTour and Eichenwald Maki 2010, 785).

292. **d**   An income statement summarizes the organization's revenue and expense transactions during the fiscal year. The income statement can be prepared at any point in time and reflects results up to that point. The income statement contains only income and expense accounts and reflects only the activity for the current fiscal year (LaTour and Eichenwald Maki 2010, 785).

293. **a** For financial reporting purposes, a fiscal year is divided into quarters (three-month periods) and months. Because the months generally end on the last calendar day, the quarters can be of slightly different duration. For example, the first quarter of a fiscal year that begins April 1 includes April, May, and June: 91 days. The second quarter of that same fiscal year includes July, August, and September: 92 days (LaTour and Eichenwald Maki 2010, 774).

294. **d** During a patient's encounter with a healthcare provider, individual services are performed and associated charges are incurred. Each charge is recorded in a subledger for the specific patient account. Because each charge represents a completed transaction, the amount of the charge becomes revenue (earned and measurable) and receivable (LaTour and Eichenwald Maki 2010, 779).

295. **d** The principle of consistency requires that the method not change over the life of the asset. Thus, the financial data are prepared in the same way from one period to the next. In fact, organizations sometimes change their choices. Consistency then requires that financial data be restated to show the effect of the change applied to previous periods (LaTour and Eichenwald Maki 2010, 775).

296. **c** Liquidity refers to the ease with which assets can be turned into cash. This is important because payroll, loan payments, and other financial obligations are typically paid in cash (LaTour and Eichenwald Maki 2010, 788–789).

297. **c** 501(c)(3) organizations are largely exempt from federal taxes but must confine their activities to the public benefit. Donations to 501(c)(3) organizations are generally tax deductible (for the donor) to the extent that no goods or services have been received in return. For that reason, charities are generally 501(c)(3) organizations and many 501(c)(6) organizations have charitable components that are separately incorporated. For example, AHIMA is a 501(c)(6) organization. The AHIMA Foundation is a 501(c)(3) organization as is the American Cancer Society. 501(c)(3) organizations may also be exempt from state sales tax under certain circumstances (LaTour and Eichenwald Maki 2010, 776–777).

298. **c** Cost–benefit feasibility is used to determine if an EHR initiative is appropriate for the organization at this time; it measures the costs associated with acquisition of hardware and software, installation, implementation, and ongoing maintenance (Amatayakul 2012, 137).

299. **c** Task structure is related to task dimension described by other theories and refers to how clearly and how well defined the task goal, procedures, and possible solutions are (LaTour and Eichenwald Maki 2010, 655).

300. **c** Charisma refers to influence by force of personality in which the leader inspires commitment, loyalty, and faith in a vision (LaTour and Eichenwald Maki 2010, 659).

301. **b** The out-group expects to be treated fairly by the leader and as long as the exchanges are viewed as fair, there is little or no conflict between the in- and out-groups; they can remain fairly stable over time (LaTour and Eichenwald Maki 2010, 656–657).

302. **b** Managers seek methods and ask how something can be done, whereas leaders seek motives and wonder why things are as they are and how they can be different (LaTour and Eichenwald Maki 2010, 647).

303. **b**   The Peter Principle refers to people who are promoted to their level of incompetency. Leaders also may find themselves in a changing organization where their previous skills are outdated. For example, some managers may have an excellent understanding of such components as the financial process, but be unable to see the broader systemic view necessary for sound strategic planning (LaTour and Eichenwald Maki 2010, 649).

304. **a**   A critical element of systems thinking is viewing an organization as an open system of interdependencies and connectedness rather than a collection of individual parts and professional enclaves. This approach sees interrelatedness as a whole and looks for patterns rather than snapshots of organizational activities and processes (Shaw and Elliott 2012, 444).

305. **c**   Early majority: This group comprises about 34 percent of the organization. Although usually not leaders, the individuals in this group represent the backbone of the organization, are deliberate in thinking and acceptance of an idea, and serve as a natural bridge between early and late adopters (LaTour and Eichenwald Maki 2010, 663).

306. **d**   Traditionally, laggards are usually the last ones to respond to innovation and make up as much as 16 percent of the organization. They are often characterized as isolated, uninformed, and mistrustful of change and change agents, but they may serve a function by keeping the organization from changing too quickly (LaTour and Eichenwald Maki 2010, 663–664).

307. **c**   Each of the adopter categories engages innovation at a different time and a different acceptance rate, as shown by the diffusion S curve. Note that during the early stages of diffusion, there is a shorter period between becoming aware of an innovation and adopting it (LaTour and Eichenwald Maki 2010, 665).

308. **c**   Some of these tools persist and have found consistent value for organizations such as strategic planning, customer relationship management, and customer market segmentation. Many common practices have been considered as fads at some time in their emergence, such as total quality management, managing by objectives, zero-based budgeting, managing by walking around, decentralizing, downsizing, and so on (LaTour and Eichenwald Maki 2010, 666).

309. **d**   An OD practitioner obtains data from the organization and involves the organization in interpreting the data and considering their implications (LaTour and Eichenwald Maki 2010, 669).

310. **a**   Several remarkably similar models of the reflective learning cycle have developed over the years. These models share the following four stages in common: doing, reflection, interpretation, and application (LaTour and Eichenwald Maki 2010, 672).

311. **c**   Strategic management is a process a leader uses for assessing a changing environment to create a vision of the future, determining how the organization fits into the anticipated environment based on its mission, vision, and knowledge of its strengths, weaknesses, opportunities, and threats, and then setting in motion a plan of action to position the organization accordingly (LaTour and Eichenwald Maki 2010, 824).

312. **a**   The trend in modern organizations is to develop each employee's leadership potential to its full capacity. This allows the employees to exercise the empowerment they are given, demonstrate their value to the organization, and perhaps participate in leadership succession in the organization (LaTour and Eichenwald Maki 2010, 647).

313. **c** The values-based organization, represented by the Servant Leadership Model, promotes 10 essential values (Greenleaf 1991; LaTour and Eichenwald Maki 2010, 660):

- *Listening* intently to clarify the will of the group as well as to hear one's own "inner voice" and seeking to discover what one's body, mind, and spirit are communicating
- *Empathize* with and understand others, assuming their good intentions, even when behaviors must be rejected
- *Healing* as a force for transformation and integration using the subtle communication of valuing the whole
- *Awareness* with courage to persist in recognizing and discussing what may be sensitive issues
- *Persuasion* rather than positional authority to build consensus and make decisions
- *Conceptualization* or vision must be balanced with daily realities
- *Foresight* requires learning lessons from the past, realities of the present, and consequences in the future using intuition
- *Stewardship* in which all stakeholders hold as their goal the greatest good for the larger society
- *Commitment* to the personal, professional, and spiritual growth of people
- *Community building* within the organization to replace what has been lost socially

314. **c** Strategic managers develop skills reflecting the implications and opportunities afforded by trends. Whether reading a journal or discussing new ideas with others, strategic managers are always testing new ideas, identifying those that have merit, and discarding those that do not. They are creating links between the trends and the value-adding actions they can take (LaTour and Eichenwald Maki 2010, 824–825).

315. **d** With organizational learning as a centerpiece, this approach unifies change management, strategy development, and leadership. In all three, we learn by observing and reflecting on the results of our experiences. This concept is best depicted in Kolb's Learning Loop (LaTour and Eichenwald Maki 2010, 826).

316. **a** Every aspect of management involves a strategic management component, as described here. With organizational learning as a centerpiece, this approach unifies change management, strategy development, and leadership. In all three, people learn by observing and reflecting on the results of experiences (LaTour and Eichenwald Maki 2010, 824).

317. **a** Change management is the process by which an organization gets to its future state. Much has been said about the need for change management to facilitate adoption of EHR, and many techniques have been used to help empower those in process assessment teams to think "outside the box" (Amatayakul 2012, 214–215).

318. **c** Work sampling is a technique of work measurement that involves using statistical probability (determined through random sample observations) to characterize the performance of the department and its work (functional) units (LaTour and Eichenwald Maki 2010, 692).

319. **b** Feedback controls are back-end processes that monitor and measure output, and then compare it to expectations and identify variations that then must be analyzed so correction action plans can be developed and implemented (LaTour and Eichenwald Maki 2010, 696).

320. **c** Customers are the people, external and internal, who receive and are affected by the work of the organization or department. They have names and needs, and are the reason(s) for the collective work of the organization (LaTour and Eichenwald Maki 2010, 699).

321. **b** In a flow process chart, an operation is symbolized with a circle, transportation with an arrow, storage with a triangle, inspection with a rectangle, and a delay with a figure resembling an uppercase D. When the symbols are connected with a line, the manager can see the actual flow of work (LaTour and Eichenwald Maki 2010, 703).

322. **b** To get the project back on track, the project manager must evaluate the available options. All these options are a variant of the variables that make up the project parameters: scope, performance, cost, and time line. A kickoff meeting is held at the beginning of a project (LaTour and Eichenwald Maki 2010, 819).

323. **b** Project risk is a situation that affects the success of a project. The risk can take many forms and be of either a technical or psychological nature and hinder the successful project outcome. For example, implementing a state-of-the-art computer system may provide leading-edge technology that sets the organization apart from its competitors. However, the availability of personnel who can provide support for new technology may be limited (LaTour and Eichenwald Maki 2010, 809).

324. **c** Before the project begins, the project manager will capture a baseline of the project schedule and work effort. The baseline is an original estimate for the project. It is captured so that the progress of the project can be compared to the original plan (LaTour and Eichenwald Maki 2010, 817).

325. **b** A project differs from the day-to-day operations of an organization. Operations are concerned with the everyday jobs needed to run the business. The personnel involved in the operational aspects of the business perform the same functions on a routine basis. This work does not end. In contrast, a project has a precise, expected result produced by defined resources within a specific time frame (LaTour and Eichenwald Maki 2010, 808).

326. **b** Every project follows a project management life cycle regardless of its size or duration. Each process in the life cycle has its own importance. Conducting a variance analysis would not be considered a part of the process (LaTour and Eichenwald Maki 2010, 811).

327. **d** There are three types of project team structure: functional, projectized, and matrixed (LaTour and Eichenwald Maki 2010, 811).

328. **b** A project plan starts with a work breakdown structure (WBS), or task list. The WBS is a hierarchical list of steps needed to complete the project. This structure provides levels that are similar to the concept of a book outline. Each level drills down to more detail. The lowest level is the task level, which is the level to which resources are assigned and work effort estimates are made (LaTour and Eichenwald Maki 2010, 814).

329. **b** A project's objectives include cost, performance, time, and scope. Project scope is the magnitude of the work to be done (LaTour and Eichenwald Maki 2010, 808).

330. **b** A project office is responsible for defining project management procedures, conducting risk analyses on projects, and mentoring project managers (LaTour and Eichenwald Maki 2010, 810).

331. **b** The project manager now should be ready to record the project objectives, scope, deliverables, expected time line, and anticipated cost in a written document. This document is known by various names. Typical names include project charter, statement of work, and project definition document or business plan (LaTour and Eichenwald Maki 2010, 813).

332. **b** One of the success factors for a project is good project communication. Several forms of project communication are used during the project: project status meetings, project status reports, issue logs, and project plans (LaTour and Eichenwald Maki 2010, 820).

333. **b** A stakeholder is anyone in the organization who is affected by the project product. Stakeholders include personnel who are on the project team, personnel whose daily work will be changed because of the project's product, and the managers and executives for those departments involved in the project. Each stakeholder has different concerns relative to the project's objectives and goals (LaTour and Eichenwald Maki 2010, 808).

334. **d** If a project manager is using project management software, the critical path for the project can be determined. The critical path is the series of specific tasks that determine the overall project duration (LaTour and Eichenwald Maki 2010, 816).

335. **b** An EHR project is not a typical IT project, and IT skills or even strong technical project management skills are less important to the EHR project manager role than vision and leadership (Amatayakul 2012, 100).

336. **a** A Gantt chart is used to show project tasks, phases, and milestones, and their start, end, and completion dates. It helps to illustrate where more than one task must be performed simultaneously. The column labeled C is the duration scheduled for the Test ADT-Lab interface for 1/12–1/16 (Amatayakul 2012, 121).

337. **c** A Gantt chart is used to illustrate project tasks, phases, and milestones, and their start, end, and completion dates. It helps to show where more than one task must be performed simultaneously. The column labeled D is showing the progress of the task "1.1 Write test scenario" (Amatayakul 2012, 121).

338. **c** Fixed costs remain the same despite changes in volume. For example, a manager's base salary does not change regardless of patient volume or other changes in activity (LaTour and Eichenwald Maki 2010, 790).

339. **b** Indirect costs are incurred by the organization in the process of providing goods or services; however, they are not specifically attributable to an individual product or service. The cost of providing security services at a hospital or clerical support at the switchboard are indirect costs with respect to patient care. Equity and liability cannot be attributed to a specific product or service. Fixed costs remain the same despite changes in volume (LaTour and Eichenwald 2010, 790).

340. **a** Variable costs are sensitive to volume. Medication is a good example—the more patients are treated, the more medication is used (LaTour and Eichenwald Maki 2010, 790).

341. **d** Direct costs are traceable to a specific good or service provided. To a hospital, the cost of a specific medication can be matched to the specific patient to whom it was administered (LaTour and Eichenwald Maki 2010, 790).

342. **b** The major components of the revenue cycle are preclaims submission activities performed by admitting and case management; claim processing activities, which is performed by multiple areas to include patient financial services and HIM coding for charge capture, Chargemaster maintenance, coding, auditing, and claims submission; accounts receivable, and claims reconciliation and collections activities performed by patient financial services (Casto and Layman 2011, 249–253).

343. **a** The Medicare Code Editor is used by the fiscal intermediary to audit claims received by hospitals to ensure that the claim contains correct information. In the claims reconciliation process, the healthcare facility used the explanation of benefits, Medicare Summary Notice, and the remittance advice to reconcile accounts (Casto and Layman 2011, 254).

344. **a** Preclaims submission activities comprise tasks and functions from the admitting and case management areas. Specifically, this portion of the revenue cycle is responsible for collecting the patient's and responsible parties' information completely and accurately for determining the appropriate financial class, educating the patient as to his or her ultimate financial responsibility for services rendered, collecting waivers when appropriate, and verifying data prior to procedures/services being performed and submitted for payment (Casto and Layman 2011, 249).

345. **c** Typical performance statistics maintained by the accounts receivable department include days in accounts receivable and aging of accounts. Aging of accounts is maintained in 30-day increments (0–30 days, 31–60 days, and so forth) (Casto and Layman 2011, 253).

346. **b** Claims-processing activities include the capture of all billable services, claim generation, and claim correction. Charge capture is a vital component of the revenue cycle (Casto and Layman 2011, 250).

347. **a** Preclaims submission activities comprise tasks and functions from the admitting and case management areas. Specifically, this portion of the revenue cycle is responsible for collecting the patient's and responsible parties' information completely and accurately for determining the appropriate financial class, educating the patient as to his or her ultimate financial responsibility for services rendered, collecting waivers when appropriate, and verifying data prior to procedures/services being performed and submitted for payment (Casto and Layman 2011, 249).

348. **d** The last component of the revenue cycle is reconciliation and collections. The healthcare facility used the explanation of benefits (EOB), Medicare summary notice (MSN), and remittance advice (RA) to reconcile accounts. EOBs and MSNs identify the amount owed by the patient to the facility. Collections can contact the patient to collect outstanding deductibles and copayments. RAs indicate rejected or denied items or claims. Facilities can review the RAs and determine where the claim error can be corrected and resubmitted for additional payment (Casto and Layman 2011, 254).

349. **b** Many facilities have internal auditing systems known as scrubbers. The auditing system runs each claim through a set of edits specifically designed for that third-party payer. The auditing system identifies data that have failed edits and flags the claim for correction (Casto and Layman 2011, 525).

350. **d** Each facility must have a policy in place for dealing with situations where records remain incomplete for an extended period. The HIM director can be given authority to declare that a record is completed for purposes of filing when a provider relocates, dies, or has an extended illness that would prevent the record from ever being completed. Every effort should be made to have a partner or physician in the same specialty area complete the charts so that coding, billing, and statistical information are available (LaTour and Eichenwald Maki 2010, 215).

351. **b** HR management activities associated with unions and collective bargaining are referred to as labor relations. Labor organizations (unions) enter into negotiations with employers on behalf of groups of employees who have elected to join a union. The negotiations relate to compensation and safety and health concerns. In a unionized environment, three laws that came into existence over a period of 25 years (1935–1960) constitute a code of practice for unions and management. HR departments pay strict attention to these three acts: National Labor Relations Act (Wagner Act), Labor-Management Relations Act (Taft–Hartley Act), Labor–Management Reporting and Disclosure Act (Landrum–Griffin Act) (Mathis and Jackson 2002; Anthony et al. 1996; LaTour and Eichenwald Maki 2010, 726–727).

352. **b** The Age Discrimination in Employment Act of 1967 protects individuals 40 years and older (Brodnik et al. 2012, 478).

353. **d** The Equal Pay Act of 1963 regulates the concept of equal pay for men and women who perform similar work requiring similar skills, effort, and responsibility under similar working conditions (Brodnik et al. 2012, 478).

354. **a** Federal legislation that makes it illegal to discriminate against individuals with disabilities in employment, public accommodations, public services, transportation, and telecommunications is the Americans with Disabilities Act of 1990 (LaTour and Eichenwald Maki 2010, 953).

355. **b** Healthcare organizations have given substantial attention to safety management since the enactment of the Occupational Safety and Health Act (OSHA) of 1970. Its intended purpose is "to assure, so far as possible, every working man or woman in the nation safe and healthful working conditions and to preserve our natural resources" (LaTour and Eichenwald Maki 2010, 726).

356. **c** Provisions of the FLSA, for example, cover minimum wage, overtime pay, child labor restrictions, and equal pay for equal work regardless of sex. Covered groups are referred to as nonexempt employees (LaTour and Eichenwald Maki 2010, 734).

357. **b** Workers' compensation is an insurance system operated by the individual states. Each state has its own law and program to provide covered workers with some protection against the costs of medical care and the loss of income resulting from work-related injuries and, in some cases, illnesses (LaTour and Eichenwald Maki 2010, 38).

358. **b** Each licensed independent contractor/practitioner who provides care under the auspices of a healthcare organization must do so in accordance with delineated clinical privileges. One of the requirements for these privileges is for the individual to carry their own professional liability insurance and therefore they are considered an independent contractor within the healthcare organization (Shaw and Elliott 2012, 294–295).

359. **a** A contract action arises when one party claims that the other party has failed to meet an obligation set forth in a valid contract. Another way to state this is that the other party has breached the contract. The resolution available is either compensation or performance of the obligation (LaTour and Eichenwald Maki 2010, 279).

360. **b** The elements of a contract must be stated clearly and specifically. A contract cannot exist unless all the following elements exist: there must be an agreement between two or more persons or entities and the agreement must include a valid offer, acceptance, and exchange of consideration (LaTour and Eichenwald Maki 2010, 278).

361. **b** The Civil Rights Act prohibits discrimination based on age, race, color, sex, religion, or national origin (Brodnik et al. 2012, 478).

362. **c** The Federal Anti-Kickback Statute (42 USC 1320a-7b[B]) establishes criminal penalties for individuals and entities that knowingly and willfully offer, pay, solicit, or receive remuneration in order to induce business for which payment may be made under any federal healthcare program including, but not limited to, kickbacks, bribes, and rebates (Brodnik et al. 2012, 435).

363. **b** Fraud in healthcare is defined independently by a number of legal authorities, but all definitions share common elements: a false representation of fact, a failure to disclose a fact that is material (relevant) to a healthcare transaction, damage to another party that reasonably relies on the misrepresentation, or failure to disclose. This situation would fall under category 2 (Brodnik et al. 2012, 430–431).

364. **c** The Family Medical Leave Act of 1993 allows employees to be granted leaves of absence for a variety of reasons including personal or family illness, pregnancy, or military service (LaTour and Eichenwald Maki 2010, 726).

365. **c** Three fundamental concepts in helping adults learn are motivation, reinforcement, and knowledge of the results. Training must be viewed as an integral part of the work environment (LaTour and Eichenwald Maki 2010, 752).

366. **d** Alternative staffing structures offer flexibility in hours, location, and job responsibilities as a method to attract and retain employees and eliminate staffing shortages. Some examples are job sharing, outsourcing, flextime, and telecommuting (LaTour and Eichenwald Maki 2010, 759–762).

367. **a** Classroom learning is still the most popular method of instruction. It enables immediate feedback and can improve communication skills. When the goal is to train a large number of employees on largely factual knowledge within a short period of time, classroom learning may be the best choice (LaTour and Eichenwald Maki 2010, 755).

368. **c** In-service education is a continuous process that builds on the basic skills learned through new employee orientation and on-the-job training. It is concerned with teaching employees specific skills and behaviors required to maintain job performance (LaTour and Eichenwald Maki 2010, 748).

369. **d** Adults like feedback on their performance. It is important to understand the concept of the learning curve. When a new task is learned, productivity may decrease while a great deal of material is actually being learned. Later, there is little new learning, but productivity may increase greatly. Either situation can be frustrating, so guidance and feedback are important to help employees understand what they have accomplished (LaTour and Eichenwald Maki 2010, 752).

370. **c** An HIM manager, who focuses exclusively on his or her own area of responsibility, whether managing a department, a service, or a project, will have a difficult time succeeding as a strategic manager. Understanding the environment provides the context for the tough decisions involved in setting direction, designing strategy, and leading change (LaTour and Eichenwald Maki 2010, 830).

371. **c** Knowledge of the internal and external environment is essential to vision and strategy formulation. An environmental assessment is conducted, which is defined as a thorough review of the internal and external conditions in which an organization operates (Jennings 2000, 39). This data-intensive process is the continuous process of gathering and analyzing intelligence about trends that are—or may be—affecting an organization and industry. IBM did not see the market demands and change in the personal home computing environment quickly enough, so their competitors were out to market ahead of them (LaTour and Eichenwald Maki 2010, 829).

372. **b** A strategy map is a tool that provides a visual representation of an organization's critical objectives and the relationships among them that drive organizational performance (Norton et al. 2000, 2). Depicting change as a road map is a useful way to help others understand the goals and the course of change (LaTour and Eichenwald Maki 2010, 833).

373. **b** Kotter asserts that "by far the biggest mistake people make when trying to change organizations is to plunge ahead without establishing a high enough sense of urgency" (1995, 59–67). Leaders may overestimate the extent to which they can force change on the organization. To increase the sense of urgency, leaders must remove or minimize the sources of complacency. Some examples of how this might be done include engaging employees, customers, and co-workers in a dialogue about change through a series of meetings; convening a project steering committee with representatives from all stakeholder groups; identifying opinion leaders and securing their support early; presenting believable stories or scenarios that illustrate the potential futures that may occur if action is not taken; and creating new vehicles for communication, such as a project newsletter (LaTour and Eichenwald Maki 2010, 837–838).

374. **b** Get new programs launched quickly by using techniques such as rapid prototyping, demonstration projects, or pilot tests. The details do not always need to be fully worked out to create visible demonstrations. The leader may not need to secure approval for full implementation as testing an approach to see its value is often accepted as a pilot (LaTour and Eichenwald Maki 2010, 838).

375. **a** Learners tend to progress only as far as they need to in order to achieve their goal. So, the best time to learn is when it is seen as useful, which has made just-in-time training popular (LaTour and Eichenwald Maki 2010, 753).

376. **b** Effective training programs begin with a needs assessment and blend an appropriate combination of methods, media, content, and activities into a curriculum that is matched to the specific education, experience, and skill level of the audience (LaTour and Eichenwald Maki 2010, 745).

377. **b** When an employee is working on his or her own, the supervisor should check the quantity and quality of the employee's work against performance standards from time to time. If the employee's performance is below standard, the training can be repeated before bad performance becomes a habit (LaTour and Eichenwald Maki 2010, 748).

378. **a** Reasons that employees stay in organizations include culture and work environment, compensation that is fair and based on performance, training and development, role of the supervisor, and growth and earning potential (LaTour and Eichenwald Maki 2010, 759).

379. **b** In the healthcare work environment, learning translates into achieving the goals of the institution, including improved job performance. The objective is for employees to develop effective work habits. To accomplish this objective, it is important to understand how employees learn and the factors that affect the learning environment (LaTour and Eichenwald 2010, 752).

380. **c** In cross-training, the employee learns to perform the jobs of many team members. This method is most useful when work teams are involved (LaTour and Eichenwald Maki 2010, 747).

381. **d** Flextime generally refers to the employee's ability to work by varying his or her starting and stopping hours around a core of midshift hours, such as 10 a.m. to 1 p.m. Depending on their position and the institution, employees may have a certain degree of freedom in determining their hours (LaTour and Eichenwald Maki 2010, 759).

382. **b** The emerging worker of the 21st century values growth over predictability, is concerned with opportunities for creativity, and understands that job security must be earned (LaTour and Eichenwald Maki 2010, 759).

383. **b** Physical safeguards have to do with protecting the environment, including ensuring applicable doors have locks that are changed when needed and that fire, flood, and other natural disaster preparedness is in place (for example, fire alarms, sprinklers, smoke detectors, raised cabinets). Other physical controls include badging and escorting visitors and other typical security functions such as patrolling the premises, logging equipment in and out, and camera-monitoring key areas. HIPAA does not provide many specifics on physical facility controls, but does require a facility security plan with the expectation that these matters will be addressed (Sayles and Trawick 2010, 315–318).

384. **b** Confidentiality is a legal ethical concept that establishes the healthcare provider's responsibility for protecting health records and other personal and private information from unauthorized use or disclosure (Brodnik et al. 2012, 5–6).

385. **c** The HIPAA Security Rule requires covered entities to ensure the confidentiality, integrity, and availability of ePHI. The Security Rule contains provisions that require covered entities to adopt administrative, physical, and technical safeguards (Brodnik et al. 2012, 272).

386. **d** The Uniform Health Care Decisions Act suggests that decision-making priority for an individual's next-of-kin be as follows: spouse, adult child, parent, adult sibling, or if no one is available who is so related to the individual, authority may be granted to "an adult who exhibited special care and concern for the individual" (Brodnik et al. 2012, 153–154).

387. **b** The HIPAA Privacy Rule states that protected health information used for purposes of treatment, payment, or healthcare operations does not require patient authorization to allow providers access, use, or disclosure. However, only the minimum necessary information needed to satisfy the specified purpose can be used or disclosed (Odom-Wesley et al. 2009, 22).

388. **b** A subpoena is a direct command that requires an individual or a representative of an organization to appear in court or to present an object to the court (Odom-Wesley et al. 2009, 57).

389. **c** Strict liability (liability without fault), means that a person is responsible for the damage and loss caused by his or her acts and omissions regardless of fault (Brodnik et al. 2012, 97).

390. **c** Generally speaking, the age of majority is 18 years old or older. This is the legal recognition that an individual is considered responsible for, and has control over, his or her actions (Brodnik et al. 2012, 149).

391. **a**   When an individual who is at or above the age of majority becomes incapacitated, either permanently or temporarily, another person should be designated to make decisions for that individual including decisions about the use and disclosure of the individual's PHI. Whoever serves as the incompetent adult's personal representative should, at minimum, hold the incompetent adult's durable power of attorney (DPOA) or durable power of attorney for healthcare decisions (DPOA-HCD) (Brodnik et al. 2012, 334).

392. **d**   The Uniform Health Care Decisions Act suggests that decision-making priority for an individual's next-of-kin be as follows: spouse, adult child, parent, adult sibling, or if no one is available who is so related to the individual, authority may be granted to "an adult who exhibited special care and concern for the individual" (Brodnik et al. 2012, 153–154).

393. **c**   Because HIPAA defers to state laws on the issue of minors, applicable state laws should be consulted regarding appropriate authorization. Generally speaking, the age of majority is 18 years old or older. This is the legal recognition that an individual is considered responsible for, and has control over, his or her actions (Brodnik et al. 2012, 149).

394. **d**   Many state laws allow a minor to be treated as an adult for drug or alcohol dependency, sexually transmitted diseases, or be given contraceptives and prenatal care without parental or legal guardian consent. This gives minors the right to treatment and access of their health records as a competent adult (Brodnik et al. 2012, 335).

395. **c**   Employers who may or may not be HIPAA-covered healthcare organizations may request patient information for a number of reasons, including family medical leave certification, return to work certification for work-related injuries, and information for company physicians. Patient authorization is required for such disclosures, except in some states the patient's employer, employer's insurer, and employer's and employee's attorneys do not need patient authorization to obtain health information for workers' compensation purposes (Brodnik et al. 2012, 336).

396. **c**   Generally, a hospital is liable to patients for the torts of its employees (including nurses and employed physicians) under the doctrine of *respondeat superior* (Latin for "let the master answer"). Also referred to as vicarious liability, under this doctrine the hospital holds itself out as responsible for the actions of its employees, provided that these individuals were acting within the scope of their employment or at the hospital's direction at the time they conducted the tortuous activity in question (Brodnik et al. 2012, 96).

397. **a**   Employees in departments such as the business office, information systems, HIM, and infection control, who are not involved directly in patient care, will vary in their need to access patient information. The HIPAA "minimum necessary" principle must be applied to determine what access employees should legitimately have to PHI (45 CFR 164.502 [b]; Brodnik et al. 2012, 336).

398. **b**   The physician would not have access to records of a patient he or she is not treating unless the physician is performing designated healthcare operations such as research, peer review, or quality management. Otherwise the physician would need to have an authorization from the patient (Brodnik et al. 2012, 336–337).

399. **a** The mental health professional can disclose information without an authorization from the patient in the following situations (Brodnik et al. 2012, 338–339):

- The patient brings up the issue of the mental or emotional condition
- The health professional performs an examination under a court order
- Involuntary commitment proceedings
- A legal "duty to warn" an intended victim when a patient threatens to harm an identifiable victim(s)
- The mental health professional believes that the patient is likely to actually harm the individual(s)

400. **b** The National Conference of Commissioners of Uniform State Laws introduced the Uniform Electronic Transactions Act. Its purpose was to make electronic transactions as enforceable as paper transactions in an effort to remove barriers to electronic commerce and increase the level of trust associated with electronic business transactions (Brodnik et al. 2012, 177).

401. **a** The law permits a presumption of consent during emergency situations regardless of whether the patient is an adult or a minor (Brodnik et al. 2012, 137).

402. **d** One of the specifications found within the consent for use and disclosure of information should state that the individual has the right to revoke the consent in writing, except to the extent that the covered entity has already taken action based on the consent. In this situation, the facility acted in good faith based on the prior authorization and therefore the release is covered under the Privacy Act (Brodnik et al. 2012, 230).

403. **a** Outcomes of quality improvement studies may be used to evaluate a physician's application for continued medical staff membership and privileges to practice. These studies are usually conducted as part of the hospital's QI activities. These review activities are considered confidential and protected from disclosure (Shaw and Elliott 2012, 429–430).

404. **c** No authorization is needed to use or disclose PHI for public health activities. Some health records contain information that is important to the public welfare. Such information must be reported to the state's public health service to ensure public safety (LaTour and Eichenwald Maki 2010, 289).

405. **a** News media personnel (and others) may have an interest in obtaining information about a public figure or celebrity who is being treated or about individuals involved in events that have cast them in the public eye. However, the media is not exempt from the restrictions imposed by the HIPAA facility directory requirement, and it is prudent for a healthcare organization to exercise even greater restraint than that mandated by the facility directory requirement with respect to the media. Parents of adult children and attorneys also need an authorization to receive patient records (Brodnik et al. 2012, 353).

406. **c** No authorization is needed to disclose PHI for public health activities. These activities include disease or injury reporting, communicable disease reporting, and other public health reporting requirements. A patient cannot refuse or limit this release of reportable disease information (LaTour and Eichenwald Maki 2010, 289).

407. **b** The Freedom of Information Act (FOIA) (1996) is a federal law through which individuals can seek access to information without authorization of the person to whom the information applies. This Act applies only to federal agencies and not the private sector. The Veterans Administration and Defense Department hospital systems are subject to this Act, but few other hospitals are. The only protection of health information held by federal agencies exists when disclosure would "constitute a clearly unwarranted invasion of personal privacy" (Miller 1986; LaTour and Eichenwald Maki 2010, 281).

408. **d** Redisclosure of health information is of significant concern to the healthcare industry. As such, the HIM professional must be alerted to state and federal statutes addressing this issue. A consent obtained by a hospital pursuant to the Privacy Rule in 45 CFR 164.506(a)(5) does not permit another hospital, healthcare provider, or clearinghouse to use or disclose information. However, the authorization content required in the Privacy Rule in 45 CFR 164.508(c)(1) must include a statement that the information disclosed pursuant to the authorization may be disclosed by the recipient and thus is no longer protected (45 CFR 164.508[c][2][iii]; LaTour and Eichenwald Maki 2010, 283).

409. **c** The Confidentiality of Alcohol and Drug Abuse Patient Records Rule is a federal rule that applies to information created for patients treated in a federally assisted drug or alcohol abuse program and specifically protects the identity, diagnosis, prognosis, or treatment of these patients. The rule generally prohibits rediscosure of health information related to this treatment except as needed in a medical emergency or when authorized by an appropriate court order or the patient's authorization (LaTour and Eichenwald Maki 2010, 281).

410. **d** Because incident reports contain facts, hospitals strive to protect their confidentiality. To ensure incident report confidentiality, no copies should be made and the original must not be filed in the health record nor removed from the files in the department responsible for maintaining them, typically risk management or QI. Also no reference to the completion of an incident report should be made in the health record. Such a reference would likely render the incident report discoverable because it is mentioned in a document that is discoverable in legal proceedings (LaTour and Eichenwald Maki 2010, 302).

411. **d** The designated record set (DRS) encompasses more information than what is normally considered part of a legal health record. A healthcare organization will need to determine which elements of the DRS will be part of its legal health record and which will not. Legal health records must meet accepted standards as defined by applicable federal regulations, state laws, and standards of accrediting agencies as well as the policies of the healthcare provider (Brodnik et al. 2012, 167–168).

412. **d** Title II of HIPAA is the most relevant title to the management of health information, containing provisions relating to the prevention of healthcare fraud and abuse and medical liability reform, as well as administrative simplification. The Privacy Rule derives from the administrative simplification provision of Title II along with the HIPAA security regulations, transactions and code set standardization requirements, unique national provider identifiers, and the enforcement rule (Brodnik et al. 2012, 216).

413. **b** A significant part of the administrative simplification process is the creation of standards for the electronic transmission of data (Brodnik et al. 2012, 216).

414. **d** Although a person or organization may, by definition, be subject to the Privacy Rule by virtue of the type of organization it is, not all information that it holds or comes into contact with is protected by the Privacy Rule. For example, the Privacy Rule has specifically excluded from its scope employment records held by the covered entity in its role as employer (45 CFR 160.103). Under this exclusion, employee health information contained within personnel files are specifically exempted from this rule (Brodnik et al. 2012, 226).

415. **d** Vendors who have a presence in a healthcare facility, agency, or organization will often have access to patient information in the course of their work. If the vendor meets the definition of a business associate (that is, it is using or disclosing an individual's PHI on behalf of the healthcare organization), a business associate agreement must be signed. If a vendor is not a business associate, employees of the vendor should sign confidentiality agreements because of their routine contact with and exposure to patient information. In this situation, Ready-Clean is not a business associate (Brodnik et al. 2012, 337).

416. **b** The Notice of Privacy Practices must explain and give examples of the uses of the patient's health information for treatment, payment, and healthcare operations, as well as other disclosures for purposes established in the regulations. If a particular use of information is not covered in the Notice of Privacy Practices, the patient must sign an authorization form specific to the additional disclosure before his or her information can be released (LaTour and Eichenwald Maki 2010, 194).

417. **b** Pursuant to the Privacy Rule, the hospital may disclose health information to law enforcement officials without authorization for law enforcement purposes for certain situations, including situations involving a crime victim. Disclosure is made in response to law enforcement officials' request for such information about an individual who is, or is suspected to be, a victim of a crime (LaTour and Eichenwald Maki 2010, 290).

418. **c** There are certain circumstances where the minimum necessary requirement does not apply, such as to healthcare providers for treatment; to the individual or his/her personal representative; pursuant to the individual's authorization to the Secretary of the HHS for investigations, compliance review, or enforcement; as required by law; or to meet other Privacy Rule compliance requirements (Brodnik et al. 2012, 239–240).

419. **a** Legislation gives a patient the right to obtain an accounting of disclosures of PHI made by the covered entity in the six years or less prior to the request date. Mandatory public health reporting is not considered part of a covered entities' operations. As a result, these disclosures must be included in an accounting of disclosures (Brodnik et al. 2012, 243–244).

420. **d** PHI may not be used or disclosed by a covered entity unless the individual who is the subject of the information authorizes the use or disclosure in writing or the Privacy Rule requires or permits such use or disclosure without the individual's authorization. In this situation, Dr. Lawson is a covered entity and thus releasing the names of his asthma patients to a pharmaceutical company requires the patients' authorization (Brodnik et al. 2012, 233).

421. **c** The Privacy Rule's general requirement is that authorization must be obtained for uses and disclosures of PHI created for research that includes treatment of the individual. Public information, deidentified data, or data that is recorded by the investigation so that the subject cannot be directly identified or identified through links are not subject to the Common Rule (Brodnik et al. 2012, 248–249).

422. **b** If a fee is assessed for a request, the fee schedule must be consulted and an invoice prepared. The fee schedule should be regularly reviewed for compliance with the HIPAA Privacy Rule and applicable state laws. A system should be developed to determine situations in which fees are not assessed, when prepayment is required, and to implement collection procedures for delinquent payments following record disclosure (Brodnik et al. 2012, 363).

423. **d** Under HIPAA, electronic protected health information (ePHI) is defined as all individually identifiable information that is created or received electronically by a healthcare provider or any other entity subject to HIPAA requirements (Brodnik et al. 2012, 272).

424. **d** Access control mechanisms are an effective means of controlling what and how users gain access to an electronic health information system. To authenticate the legitimate user of ePHI, the user must be assigned a unique identifier. Because of the public nature of the log-on, there is a need to authenticate the identity of the user, commonly with a password. Password systems allow for easily remembered log-ons that are hard to crack (Brodnik et al. 2012, 278–279).

425. **b** A covered entity is any provider of medical or other healthcare services or supplies who transmits any health information in electronic form in connection with a transaction for which HHS has adopted a standard (Brodnik et al. 2012, 226).

426. **c** The three methods of two-factor authentication are something you know, such as a password or PIN; something you have, such as an ATM card, token, or swipe, smart card; and something you are, such as a biometric fingerprint, voice scan, iris, or retinal scan (Brodnik et al. 2012, 305).

427. **a** Because of overlap in topics and outlines, combining HIPAA privacy and security training is a recommended process for workforce training (Brodnik et al. 2012, 290–291).

428. **d** Because minors are, as a general rule, legally incompetent and unable to make decisions regarding use and disclosure of their own healthcare information, this authority belongs to the minor's parent(s) or legal guardian(s) unless an exception applies. Generally, only one parent's signature is required to authorize the use or disclosure of a minor's PHI. In this case, the parents are the legal guardians of the minor (Brodnik et al. 2012, 334).

429. **c** Most states require healthcare personnel to report suspected abuse of specified classes of individuals such as children, the elderly, and other vulnerable categories of individuals such as the mentally disabled (Brodnik et al. 2012, 173).

430. **d** A subpoena instructing the recipient to bring documents and other records with himself or herself to a deposition or to court is a subpoena *duces tecum* (Brodnik et al. 2012, 37).

431. **d** The Business Record Exception is the rule under which a record is determined to not be hearsay if it was made at or near the time by, or from information transmitted by, a person with knowledge; it was kept in the course of a regularly conducted business activity; and it was the regular practice of that business activity to make the record (Brodnik et al. 2012, 71).

432. **c** As the healthcare industry moves toward EHRs and key evidence contained in other electronic documents such as e-mails, a new legal term has evolved: e-discovery. The US Supreme Court recently amended the Federal Rules of Civil Procedures to address the discovery of electronic records, creating a new paradigm with respect to the production of documents as a discovery method (Brodnik et al. 2012, 57–59).

433. **c** Sometimes an individual's consent to a medical exam or intervention is not freely given, but is instead ordered by a court or through some other governmental action. This situation most often arises when the welfare of the public outweighs the individual's right to withhold consent (Brodnik et al. 2012, 140).

434. **a** Elements of a valid subpoena commonly include the name of the court from which the subpoena was issued; the caption of action (the names of the plaintiff and defendant); assigned case docket number; date, time, and place of requested appearance; the information commanded, such as testimony or the specific documents sought in a subpoena *duces tecum* and the form in which that information is to be produced; the name of the issuing attorney; the name of the recipient being directed to disclose the records; and the signature or stamp of the court. The subpoena does not need to be signed by both the plaintiff and the defendant (Brodnik et al. 2012, 38).

435. **b** *Darling v. Charleston Community Memorial Hospital* (1965) is a landmark case that established a hospital's responsibility for patient care. Touching directly on quality are the issues of the facility's responsibility to have effective methods of credentialing in place and effective mechanisms for continuing medical evaluation. The facility is responsible for knowing whether the care it provides meets acceptable standards of care (LaTour and Eichenwald Maki 2010, 522).

436. **c** One of the five categories of health informatics standards are structure and content standards which establish clear descriptions of the data elements to be collected (Odom-Wesley et al. 2009, 310).

437. **d** Advance directives include such items as living wills and statements of a patient's wishes in case of a critical illness, such as life support, ventilator support, and food and hydration. The admissions staff is required by law to ask patients whether they have established advance directives and to inform patients that they have the right to accept or refuse medical treatment (Odom-Wesley et al. 2009, 99).

438. **d** ASTM Standard E1384-02a identifies the content and structure for EHRs. The scope of this standard covers all types of healthcare services including acute-care hospitals, ambulatory care, skilled nursing facilities, home healthcare, and specialty environments (LaTour and Eichenwald Maki 2010, 179).

439. **b** LOINC is a well-accepted set of terminology standards that provide a standard set of universal names and codes for identifying individual laboratory and clinical results (LaTour and Eichenwald Maki 2010, 181).

440. **c** Health Level 7 (HL7) is an organization that develops standards related to healthcare delivery (Odom-Wesley et al. 2009, 33).

441. **c** The Minimum Data Set for Long-term Care is a federally mandated standard assessment form used to collect demographic and clinical data on nursing home residents. It consists of a core set of screening and assessment elements based on common definitions. To meet federal requirements, long-term care facilities must complete an MDS for every resident at the time of admission and at designated reassessment points throughout the resident's stay (LaTour and Eichenwald Maki 2010, 166–168).

442. **c** The Centers for Disease Control and Prevention (CDC), through its National Immunization Program, provides funding for some population-based immunization registries. The CDC has identified 12 minimum functional standards for population-based immunization registries (LaTour and Eichenwald Maki 2010, 337).

443. **d** Digital imaging and communication in medicine (DICOM) is a standard that promotes a digital image communications format and picture archive and communications systems for use with digital images. In order for a radiology department to transmit images, they must implement the DICOM standards (LaTour and Eichenwald Maki 2010, 181).

444. **a** Deemed status means accrediting bodies such as the Joint Commission or AOA can survey facilities for compliance with the Medicare Conditions of Participation for hospitals instead of government (Odom-Wesley et al. 2009, 291).

445. **d** National Committee on Vital and Health Statistics has developed the initial efforts at creating standardized data sets for use in different types of healthcare settings, including acute care, ambulatory care, long-term care, and home care (LaTour and Eichenwald Maki 2010, 165).

446. **d** Hospitals and other healthcare facilities develop health record retention policies to ensure that health records comply with all applicable state and federal regulations and accreditation standards (Odom-Wesley et al. 2009, 67).

447. **a** The Medicare Conditions of Participation (2006) require that the patient's principal diagnosis be documented by the attending physician in the patient's health record no more than 30 days after discharge (Odom-Wesley et al. 2009, 201).

448. **a** Qualitative analysis is a review of the health record to ensure clinical protocols are met and determine the adequacy of entries documenting the quality of care (Odom-Wesley et al. 2009, 248).

449. **a** The Joint Commission requires accredited hospitals and other healthcare facilities to implement systems for identifying and addressing sentinel events. A sentinel event is described as an unexpected occurrence involving death or serious physical or psychological injury, or the risk thereof (Odom-Wesley et al. 2009, 303).

450. **b** Long-term, acute-care hospitals are required to have physician acknowledgment statements signed and dated from the attending physician at the initial time of credentialing for admitting privileges just as is required for short-term, acute-care hospitals (Odom-Wesley et al. 2009, 351).

451. **c** State laws, CMS regulations, and other federal regulations, accreditation standards, and facility policies and procedures must also be reviewed when establishing a retention schedule. The HIM professional must adhere to the strictest time limit if the recommended retention period varies among different laws and regulations (LaTour and Eichenwald Maki 2010, 221).

452. **b** In the case of a stillborn infant, a separate patient record is not created—information is recorded in the mother's delivery record (LaTour and Eichenwald Maki 2010, 202).

453. **c** Emergency patients must be made aware of their rights. Transfer and acceptance policies and procedures must be delineated to ensure facilities comply with the Emergency Medical Treatment and Active Labor Act (EMTALA) and state regulations regarding transfers (LaTour and Eichenwald Maki 2010, 202).

454. **a** Transfer and acceptance policies and procedures must be delineated to ensure that facilities comply with the Emergency Medical Treatment and Active Labor Act (EMTALA) and state regulations regarding transfers. The hospital must stabilize the medical emergency by ensuring an airway and ventilation, controlling hemorrhage, and stabilizing or splinting fractures before a patient can be transferred. Appropriate transfer means that the receiving hospital agrees to receive the patient and provide appropriate medical treatment. Records must be provided to the receiving hospital and the patient or responsible person must understand the medical necessity of the transfer (LaTour and Eichenwald Maki 2010, 202).

455. **c** The Joint Commission specifies that the number of delinquent records cannot exceed 50 percent of the average number of discharges (LaTour and Eichenwald Maki 2010, 215).

456. **d** Some facilities use autoauthentication even though the Joint Commission does not approve it because evidence cannot be provided that the physician actually reviewed and approved each dictated report (LaTour and Eichenwald Maki 2010, 213).

457. **a** When a facility or practice is closed or sold, its health records are transferred to the successor provider, meaning the entity or individual that purchases the facility. In ambulatory care settings or physician offices, patients are informed of their options to transfer their records to another provider or choice before their health records are transferred to the successor provider (LaTour and Eichenwald Maki 2010, 222).

458. **b** Federal administrative agencies are required to make agency rules, opinions, orders, records, and proceedings available to the public (Administrative Procedures Act 552). The publication used to accomplish this is the *Federal Register,* which is issued by the US Governmental Printing Office every business day (LaTour and Eichenwald Maki 2010, 273).

459. **b** The emergency operations plan is practiced twice a year in response either to an actual disaster or to a planned drill. Exercises should stress the limits of the organization's emergency management system to assess preparedness capabilities and performance when systems are stressed (Shaw and Elliott 2012, 250–262).

460. **a** The Commission on Accreditation of Rehabilitation Facilities (CARF) is a private, not-for-profit organization committed to developing and maintaining practical, customer-focused standards to help organizations measure and improve the quality, value, and outcomes of behavioral health and medical rehabilitation programs. CARF accreditation is based on an organization's commitment to continually enhance the quality of its services and programs and to focus on customer satisfaction (Shaw and Elliott 2012, 343–344).

Exam 1 Answers

1. **a** Transfer or referral forms provide document communication between care-givers in multiple healthcare settings. It is important that a patient's treatment plan be consistent as the patient moves through the healthcare delivery system (Odom-Wesley et al. 2009, 131).

2. **c** The chief complaint or reason for the visit is the nature and duration of the symptoms that caused the patient's illness (Odom-Wesley et al. 2009, 331).

3. **a** Discrete data are whole numbers that may or may not be related, so a bar graph is the best data display tool to use (Shaw and Elliott 2012, 48).

4. **a** Clustering is the practice of coding/charging one or two middle levels of service codes exclusively under the philosophy, that, although some will be higher and some lower, the charges will average out over an extended period (Kuehn 2012, 347).

5. **c** A nomenclature is a system of names or terms used for a particular discipline created to facilitate communication by eliminating ambiguity. The terms classification and nomenclature are often used interchangeably, but they are different. A classification system categorizes and aggregates, while a nomenclature supports detailed descriptions (LaTour and Eichenwald Maki 2010, 348).

6. **a** Clinical information is data that are related to the patient's diagnosis or treatment in a healthcare facility (Odom-Wesley et al. 2009, 55).

7. **c** Coded data are data that have been translated into a standard nomenclature or classification so they can be aggregated, analyzed, and compared. To facilitate the analysis of large amounts of information, coded data frequently are grouped into meaningful categories. The categories may be as simple as M for male and F for female or as extensive as those used to code diagnoses and procedures. The grouping may be simplistic, as in age range, or as complex as the methodology used in prospective payment systems (LaTour and Eichenwald Maki 2010, 89).

8. **b** Licensure is required prior to a hospital's opening and providing medical services (Odom-Wesley et al. 2009, 48).

9. **c** The principal function of the health record is to serve as the repository of clinical documentation relevant to the care of individual patients (Odom-Wesley et al. 2009, 40).

10. **d** Financial data includes details about the patient's occupation, employer, and insurance coverage and are collected at the time of treatment (Odom-Wesley et al. 2009, 42).

11. **c** The Subjective, Objective, Assessment, Plan (SOAP) notes are part of the problem-oriented medical records (POMR) approach most commonly used by physicians and other healthcare professionals. SOAP notes are intended to improve the quality and continuity of client services by enhancing communication among healthcare professionals (Odom-Wesley et al. 2009, 217).

12. **a** Outpatient coding guidelines do not allow coding of possible conditions as a diagnosis for the patient. Do not code diagnoses documented as "probable," "suspected," "questionable," "rule out," or "working diagnosis," or other similar terms indicating uncertainty. Rather, code the condition(s) to the highest degree of certainty for that encounter/visit, such as symptoms, signs, abnormal test results, or other reason for the visit (Kuehn 2012, 32).

13. **d** The two purposes of uniform data sets are as follows: they ensure the same types of data are collected for the patient, and they provide standardized definitions of the data to be collected (Odom-Wesley et al. 2009, 94).

14. **a** Case-mix analysis is a method of grouping patients according to a predefined set of characteristics (Odom-Wesley et al. 2009, 43).

15. **d** The MDS is the first component of the RAI and is used to collect information about the resident's risk factors and to plan the ongoing care and treatment of the resident in the long-term care facility (Odom-Wesley et al. 2009, 368).

16. **a**   RAPs form a critical link to decisions about care planning and provide guidance on how to synthesize assessment information within a comprehensive assessment (Odom-Wesley et al. 2009, 369).

17. **c**   Home health agencies are expected to conduct an assessment that accurately reflects the patient's current health status and includes information to establish and monitor a plan of care. The plan of care must be reviewed and updated at least every 60 days or as often as the severity of the patient's condition requires (Odom-Wesley et al. 2009, 388).

18. **d**   If the patient is admitted in withdrawal or if withdrawal develops after admission, the withdrawal code is designated as the principal diagnosis. The code for substance abuse/dependence is listed second (Schraffenberger 2012, 148).

19. **a**   The anemia would be sequenced first based on principal diagnosis guidelines (Schraffenberger 2012, 66).

20. **d**   The patient was admitted for the senile cataract and the procedures were completed for that condition. This follows the UHDDS guidelines for principal diagnosis selection. There is also no causal relationship given between the diabetes and the cataract, so 250.50 would be incorrect (Schraffenberger 2012, 66, 124).

21. **d**   The patient was admitted for COPD, so this is listed as the principal diagnosis. Code 491.21 is used when the medical record includes documentation of COPD with acute exacerbation. ICD-9-CM presumes a cause-and-effect relationship and classifies chronic kidney disease with hypertension as hypertensive chronic kidney disease, assign code 403.90; however, the code also at category 403 directs the coder to also code the chronic renal failure, 585.9 (Schraffenberger 2012, 210, 223).

22. **c**   The closed reduction of the fracture is coded first following principal procedure guidelines. The laceration repair is also coded. When more than one classification of wound repair is performed, all codes are reported, with the code for the most complicated procedure listed first (Kuehn 2012, 27–29).

23. **c**   A bronchoscopy with brushings and washings is considered a diagnostic bronchoscopy and not a biopsy. Code 31623 specifies brushings, and 31622 is selected for washings (Kuehn 2012, 136–137).

24. **d**   Modifiers are appended to the code to provide more information or alert the payer that a payment change is required. Modifier –55 is used to identify that the physician provided only postoperative care services for a particular procedure (Kuehn 2012, 295).

25. **b**   Begin at main term Destruction, hemorrhoid, thermal. Thermal includes infrared coagulation (Kuehn 2012, 20, 27).

26. **b**   The second process of data quality management is collection, which is the process by which data elements are gathered (Odom-Wesley et al. 2009, 385).

27. **b**   The coding professional's first responsibility is to ensure the accuracy of coded data. To this end, AHIMA has established a code of professional ethics by which coders must abide (LaTour and Eichenwald Maki 2010, 399).

28. **c** These procedures have been unbundled. Unbundling is the practice of coding services separately that should be coded together as a package because all the parts are included within one code and, therefore, one price. Unbundling done deliberately to obtain a higher reimbursement is a misrepresentation of services and can be considered fraud (Kuehn 2012, 347).

29. **d** Medicare drug benefit was created by the Medicare Modernization Act (MMA) and implemented on January 1, 2006. The program offers outpatient drug coverage provided by private prescriptions drug plans and Medicare Advantage (Casto and Layman 2011, 85).

30. **d** Workers' compensation is a payer that pays for healthcare services due to work-related incidents (Casto and Layman 2011, 6).

31. **b** Episode-of-care reimbursement is a healthcare payment method in which providers receive one lump sum for all the services they provide related to a condition or disease (Casto and Layman 2011, 10).

32. **b** Capitated rate is a method of payment for health services in which the third-party payer reimburses providers a fixed, per capita amount for a period. *Per capita* means per head or per person. A common phrase in capitated contracts is per member per month (PMPM). The PMPM is the amount of money paid each month for each individual enrolled in the health insurance plan. Capitation is characteristic of HMOs (Casto and Layman 2011, 10).

33. **b** The pre-existing period is a period of time during which healthcare insurance plans may deny coverage for certain conditions. In this situation, that patient was not covered for 12 months by her previous employer, so she will have a reduced waiting period of up to four months for any pre-existing conditions (Casto and Layman 2011, 69–70).

34. **b** The labor portion is adjusted for the wage index of the geographic area. This adjustment provides for the variations in wages across the country. For example, the cost of living is higher in San Francisco, CA, than in the state of Wyoming, so consequently the salaries are higher too. Therefore, the wage index for San Francisco, CA, is higher than Wyoming's (Casto and Layman 2011, 144).

35. **a** The explanation of benefits (EOB) is a report from a third-party payer that is sent from a healthcare insurer to the policy holder and provider. The EOB describes how the claim was processed by the healthcare insurer. It will include the actual charge for the service, the allowable amount under the payer agreement, the amount paid to the provider, and the remaining balance (if any) that the policy holder is obligated to pay (Casto and Layman 2011, 73–74).

36. **d** Integrated delivery system is a term referring to the collaboration integration of healthcare providers (Casto and Layman 2011, 107–108).

37. **c** Running a mock query would be part of application testing that ensures every function of the new computer system works. Application testing also ensures the system meets the functional requirements and other required specifications in the RFP or contract (Sayles and Trawick 2010, 142).

38. **b** A pie chart is an easily understood chart in which the sizes of the slices of the pie show the proportional contribution of each part. Pie charts can be used to show the component parts of a single group or variable. In this case, the intent is to show the proportion of each payer to the whole payer mix (LaTour and Eichenwald Maki 2010, 446–448).

39. **b**   An incidence rate is used to compare the frequency of disease in populations. Populations are compared using rates instead of raw numbers because rates adjust for differences in population size. The incidence rate is the probability or risk of illness in a population over a period of time (LaTour and Eichenwald Maki 2010, 442).

40. **d**   A notifiable disease is one for which regular, frequent, and timely information on individual cases is considered necessary to prevent and control disease. The list of notifiable diseases varies over time and by state, however, HIV/AIDS would be a notifiable disease anywhere (LaTour and Eichenwald Maki 2010, 443).

41. **c**   A table is an orderly arrangement of values that groups data into rows and columns. It should have specific, understandable headings for every column and row (LaTour and Eichenwald Maki 2010, 445).

42. **c**   This type of data would be found on a dashboard report provided to the hospital's board of directors. The measures show a dramatic change in patient safety issues at this organization. The board would now need to investigate to determine why these changes occurred (Shaw and Elliott 2012, 322–323).

43. **d**   The patient meets the severity of illness with the vaginal bleeding but does not meet intensity of service because the surgery is not being performed as an inpatient. She would not meet the admission criteria provided (Shaw and Elliott 2012, 113, 120).

44. **c**   An infection that was present in the patient before he or she was admitted to the facility is called community-acquired. In this situation, measles has an incubation period of at least 14 days, so it was community-acquired (Shaw and Elliott 2012, 162).

45. **c**   Benchmarking is the systematic comparison of the products, services, and outcomes of an organization with those of a similar organization. Benchmarking comparisons also can be made using regional and national standards or some combination (Shaw and Elliott 2012, 16).

46. **d**   An HIM professional can be involved in quality management in a variety of ways, including: collecting data and information; organizing, interpreting, and reporting data in a meaningful way; knowing data sources; and understanding clinical processes. In addition to the preceding ways of providing direct quality management involvement, the HIM professional role includes bringing basic guiding principles of solid information management to the attention of his or her organization. HIM professionals however do not make judgments about the quality of care given; this is left to the clinical staff (LaTour and Eichenwald Maki 2010, 520).

47. **a**   An indicator is a performance measure that enables healthcare organizations to monitor a process to determine whether it is meeting process requirements. Monitoring blood sugars on admission and discharge is an indicator of the quality of care delivered to the diabetes patient during the stay (Shaw and Elliott 2012, 118–119).

48. **b**   Universal protocol incorporates the principles of eliminating wrong-site, wrong-procedure, and wrong-person surgery. The steps involved in this protocol include preoperative verification process, marking of the operative site, and a "time-out" before starting any procedure (LaTour and Eichenwald Maki 2010, 529).

49. **d**   Surveys should be written at the reading level of the respondents, consistent formats should be used, all possible responses should be mutually exclusive, and terminology that the respondents understand should be incorporated. This survey used inconsistent formatting and did not have mutually exclusive responses in the age question (Shaw and Elliott 2012, 98–100).

50. **b** The employee turnover rate is over the internal benchmark for this hospital, so a performance improvement (PI) team should be formed to determine what the causes for this increase were. This increase in the turnover rate represents an opportunity for improvement (Shaw and Elliott 2012, 8).

51. **b** One purpose of risk management is to investigate a medical error that resulted in the death of a patient (Odom-Wesley et al. 2009, 46).

52. **b** The average length of stay (ALOS) is calculated from the total LOS. The total LOS divided by the number of patients discharged is the ALOS. Using the data provided, the ALOS for the 9 patients discharged on April 1st is 6 days (54 / 9) (LaTour and Eichenwald Maki 2010, 429).

53. **c** The purpose and responsibilities of the IRB are to protect the rights and welfare of human subjects as they engage in research activities. The IRB must abide by the regulations as listed in 45 CFR 46.111 and 21 CFR 56.111. The IRB must first determine if research is being conducted and then determine if human subjects are being protected (LaTour and Eichenwald Maki 2010, 564).

54. **a** Reporting statistics for a healthcare facility is similar to reporting statistics for a community. Rates for healthcare facilities are reported as per 100 cases or percent; a community rate is reported as per 1,000, 10,000, or 100,000 people (LaTour and Eichenwald Maki 2010, 424).

55. **d** Performance measurement is the process of comparing the outcomes of an organization, work unit, or employee to pre-established performance standards. The results of performance measurement are usually expressed as percentages, rates, ratios, averages, or other quantitative assessment. It is used to assess quality and productivity in clinical and administrative services. (LaTour and Eichenwald Maki 2010, 696–698).

56. **b** The mean is sensitive to extreme measures. That is, it is strongly influenced by outliers (LaTour and Eichenwald Maki 2010, 454–455).

57. **b** Strategic IS planning is the process of identifying and prioritizing IS needs based on the healthcare organization's mission and strategic goals (LaTour and Eichenwald Maki 2010, 145).

58. **c** Although there are many different models of the SDLC, all generally include a variation of the following four phases: analysis, design, implementation, and maintenance and evaluation. Alignment and improvement are not one of the four phases of the SDLC (LaTour and Eichenwald Maki 2010, 148).

59. **a** In the analysis phase of the SDLC, it is important to examine the current system and identify opportunities for improvement or enhancement. Even though an initial assessment would be completed as part of the strategic information planning process, the analysis phase of the SDLC involves a more extensive evaluation (LaTour and Eichenwald Maki 2010, 149).

60. **a** In an ASP model, there is much less upfront capital outlay and fewer IT staff required in-house. In fact, the ASP acquisition strategy may be considered essentially a financing model (Amatayakul 2012, 374).

61. **c** As the senior leadership team engages in strategic planning discussions, they should ensure that IS leadership is also engaged in these discussions. In particular, they should examine the organization's view of the role that IS technology will play in the organization's future (LaTour and Eichenwald Maki 2010, 146).

62. **b**   Network administrators are involved in installing, configuring, managing, monitoring, and maintaining network applications. They are responsible for supporting the network infrastructure and controlling user access (LaTour and Eichenwald Maki 2010, 154).

63. **c**   Conversion to a new system often requires major changes in the workflow and organizational structure. These changes in workflow patterns, noise, space, telephone lines, and electrical power should all take place as part of the implementation phase of the SDLC (LaTour and Eichenwald Maki 2010, 150).

64. **d**   Switch is a service that enables the exchange of information across multiple independent enterprises that have unilateral independent exchange data and in which there is no access to personal health information (Amatayakul 2012, 592).

65. **b**   The entity-relationship diagram (ERD) was developed to depict relational database structures. It can be used to depict conceptual-level models for any type of database but would only be used to model a relational database at the logical level (Amatayakul 2012, 268–269).

66. **b**   A many-to-many relationship occurs only in a data model developed at the conceptual level. In this case, the relationship between PATIENTS and CONSULTING PHYSICIANS is many-to-many. For each instance of PATIENT, there could be many instances of CONSULTING PHYSICIAN because patients can be seen by more than one consulting physician. For each instance of CONSULTING PHYSICIAN, there could be many PATIENTS because the physician sees many patients (Sayles and Trawick 2010, 96–97).

67. **a**   A virtual private network (VPN) is a special kind of wide area network (WAN) that uses a private tunnel through the Internet as the transport medium between locations rather than privately owned cable or leased lines. A VPN reduces networking costs significantly because much of the maintenance is performed by an Internet service provider (Amatayakul 2012, 298–299).

68. **b**   The primary key (PK) for PATIENT, PATIENT_MRN, is repeated in VISIT, as is the PK for CLINIC, CLINIC_ID. These keys are called foreign keys (FK) in the VISIT table. Foreign keys allow relationships between tables. By having the foreign keys in VISIT, the information in PATIENT and CLINIC is linked through the VISIT table (LaTour and Eichenwald Maki 2010, 129–130).

69. **b**   The data dictionary may also control if a mask is used and if so, what form it takes. The social security number of 123456789 could be entered and it appears in the system as 123-45-6789. The use of the mask tells the database what format to use to display the number (Sayles and Trawick 2010, 94).

70. **c**   HL7 is a standards development organization accredited by the American National Standards Institute that addresses issues at the seventh, or application level, of healthcare system interconnections (LaTour and Eichenwald Maki 2010, 178).

71. **b**   When complex analyses are to be performed on data, a clinical data warehouse (CDW) may be the more appropriate database structure to use. Data warehouses are designed to receive data (often as an extraction of data from a repository) and perform complex, analytical processes on the data (LaTour and Eichenwald Maki 2010, 242).

72. **b**   A universal chart order system is one in which the patient health record is kept in the same format/order while the patient is in the facility and after discharge (LaTour and Eichenwald Maki 2010, 212).

73. **c**   Aggregate data are used to develop information about groups of patients (LaTour and Eichenwald Maki 2010, 164).

74. **a**   Healthcare Cost and Utilization Project (HCUP) uses data collected at the state level from either claims data from the UB-04 or discharge-abstracted data, including UHDDS items reported by individual hospitals and, in some cases, by freestanding ambulatory care centers, regardless of payers (LaTour and Eichenwald Maki 2010, 341).

75. **c**   A logic-based encoder prompts the user through a variety of questions and choices based on the clinical terminology entered. The coder selects the most accurate code for a service or condition and any possible complications or comorbidities (LaTour and Eichenwald Maki 2010, 400).

76. **a**   An audit trail is a chronological set of computerized records that provides evidence of information system activity (log-ins and log-outs, file accesses) used to determine security violations (LaTour and Eichenwald Maki 2010, 79).

77. **b**   It is vitally important to be able to compare data for outcomes measurement, quality improvement, resource utilization, best practices, and medical research. These tasks can be accomplished only when healthcare has a common terminology that is easily integrated into the EHR (LaTour and Eichenwald Maki 2010, 348).

78. **a**   Role-based access control (RBAC) is a control system in which access decisions are based on the roles of individual users as part of an organization (Brodnik et al. 2012, 304).

79. **c**   As important as firewalls are to the overall security of health information systems, they cannot protect a system from all types of attacks. Many viruses, for example, can hide within documents that will not be stopped by a firewall (Brodnik et al. 2012, 311–312).

80. **b**   An audit trail is a record that shows who accessed a computer system, when it was accessed, and what operations were performed. These can be categorized as follows: individual accountability, reconstructing electronic events, problem monitoring, and intrusion detection (Brodnik et al. 2012, 307–308).

81. **d**   The data elements in a patient's automated laboratory order, result, or demographic or financial information system are coded and alphanumeric. Their fields are predefined and limited. In other words, the type of data is discrete, and the format of these data is structured (LaTour and Eichenwald Maki 2010, 52).

82. **b**   Some diagnostic image data are based on analog, photographic films, such as an analog chest x-ray. These analog films must be digitally scanned, using film digitizers, to digitize the data (LaTour and Eichenwald Maki 2010, 52).

83. **d**   Natural language processing technology considers sentence structure (syntax), meaning (semantics), and context to accurately process and extract free-text data, including speech data for application purposes. When one talks at natural speed without pausing between words, the natural language voice bytes are, indeed, processed by this technology (LaTour and Eichenwald Maki 2010, 54).

84. **b** The EHR extension model of the PHR extends the EHR into cyberspace so an authorized patient can access the provider's record and check the record's content. Often this model allows an authorized patient to extract data from the healthcare provider's record. The record is still maintained by the provider but is available to the patient in an online format (LaTour and Eichenwald Maki 2010, 76).

85. **d** Electronic data interchange (EDI) allows the transfer (incoming and outgoing) of information directly from one computer to another by using flexible, standard formats. The billing function was one of the first to utilize this technology in healthcare (LaTour and Eichenwald Maki 2010, 56–57).

86. **c** Computer output laser disk/enterprise report management (COLD/ERM) technology electronically stores, manages, and distributes documents that are generated in a digital format and whose output data are report-formatted and print-stream originated. COLD/ERM technology not only electronically stores the report-formatted documents but also distributes them with fax, e-mail, web, and traditional hard-copy print processes (LaTour and Eichenwald Maki 2010, 59–60).

87. **a** Application service providers (ASPs) are service firms that deliver, manage, and remotely host ("remote hosting" being a common term associated with ASPs) standardized (prepackaged) applications software through centralized servers via a network, not exclusively, but more commonly, the Internet (Amatayakul 2012, 373–374).

88. **b** The master patient index (MPI) is a database of patients and individuals for which healthcare services are delivered or completed (Odom-Wesley et al. 2009, 78).

89. **a** A digital signature is a digitized version of a handwritten signature. The author of the documentation signs his or her name on a pen pad, and the signature is automatically converted to a digital signature that is affixed to the electronic document (Odom-Wesley et al. 2009, 263).

90. **c** Intranets link every employee within an organization via an easy-to-navigate, comprehensive network devoted to internal business operations. Intranets are designed to enhance communication among an organization's internal employees and facilities. Web-based intranets offer better security than use of the "public" Internet and are less expensive to implement and easier to use than most private networks of proprietary mail and messaging software products (LaTour and Eichenwald Maki 2010, 62–63).

91. **c** Healthcare informatics is the field of information science concerned with the management of all aspects of health data and information through the application of computers and computer technologies (LaTour and Eichenwald Maki 2010, 48).

92. **b** Administrative safeguards are people-focused and include requirements such as training and assignment of an individual responsible for security (Sayles and Trawick 2010, 301).

93. **a** The external change agent has the advantage of providing a fresh, outside view as well as having the knowledge base to compare performance across organizations. Not having direct connections to the organization, he or she usually feels more comfortable challenging norms and culture, questioning unusual or unfair practices, and generally noting events that others may be reluctant to comment on. Being from the outside, he or she may be seen as having new skills and being more objective, or at least less biased than an internal agent (LaTour and Eichenwald Maki 2010, 668).

94. **a** According to the Joint Commission, the physical exam must be completed within 24 hours of admission (Odom-Wesley et al. 2009, 353).

95. **d** Provisions of the FLSA, for example, cover minimum wage, overtime pay, child labor restrictions, and equal pay for equal work regardless of sex. Covered groups are referred to as nonexempt employees (LaTour and Eichenwald Maki 2010, 734).

96. **b** Flextime generally refers to the employee's ability to work by varying his or her starting and stopping hours around a core of midshift hours, such as 10 a.m. to 1 p.m. Depending on their position and the institution, employees may have a certain degree of freedom in determining their hours. For example, an employee may be given flexibility to start any time between 6 a.m. and 8 a.m. and leave after having worked seven hours (LaTour and Eichenwald Maki 2010, 759).

97. **b** Appreciative inquiry is based on the belief that whatever is needed in organizational renewal already exists somewhere in the organization. It is a solution-oriented approach that seeks to identify where the change already works and how it can be amplified and transferred elsewhere in the organization (LaTour and Eichenwald Maki 2010, 670).

98. **c** The idea of the "glass barrier" or "glass ceiling" was originally coined by Carol Hymowitz and Timothy Schellhardt in a 1986 *Wall Street Journal* article. The term refers to an unofficial barrier imposed to prevent certain groups, especially women, from progressing to higher levels of management in organizations. Since its introduction, the concept has raised awareness of the role and contribution of women and the importance of diversifying the workforce (LaTour and Eichenwald Maki 2010, 661).

99. **d** First calculate the number of productive hours in a day: 88% $\times$ 8 hours = 7.04 hours/day. Then divide the 1,000 charts/7 hours = 142.9 or 143 charts / hour for the three filers (LaTour and Eichenwald Maki 2010, 690).

100. **c** Many employers pay a slightly higher hourly wage to employees who work less desirable shifts (evening, night, weekend). This is referred to as shift differential (LaTour and Eichenwald Maki 2010, 685).

101. **c** A position (job) description outlines the work to be performed by a specific employee or group of employees with the same responsibilities. Position descriptions generally consist of three parts: a summary of the position's requirements and purpose, its functions, and the qualifications needed to perform the job. Position descriptions also include the official title of the job (LaTour and Eichenwald Maki 2010, 727–729).

102. **a** Standards that are measurable and relevant to an employee's overall performance are helpful in setting clear expectations. They also are useful in providing constructive feedback (LaTour and Eichenwald Maki 2010, 689).

103. **b** Most communication errors are between healthcare professionals in different disciplines (Gardner 2003). In addition, the hierarchical nature of most healthcare organizations is a source of miscommunication. As messages travel through several layers and channels, information is added, dropped out, or modified (LaTour and Eichenwald Maki 2010, 640).

104. **a** Mentoring is a form of coaching. A mentor is a senior employee who works with employees early in their careers, giving them advice on developing skills and career options. Several employees may be assigned as protégés to the mentor, but contact is usually one-on-one. Through the mentoring relationship, employees have an advisor with whom they can solve problems, analyze and learn from mistakes, and celebrate successes. Many organizations have formal mentoring programs where protégés are matched with potential mentors. Other managers voluntarily offer to work with up-and-coming employees (LaTour and Eichenwald Maki 2010, 764).

105. **d** After employees have been recruited and selected, the first step is to introduce them to the organization and their immediate work setting and functions. New employee orientation includes a group of activities that introduce the employee to the organization's mission, policies, rules, and culture; the department or workgroup; and the specific job he or she will be performing (LaTour and Eichenwald Maki 2010, 743).

106. **a** Fee-for-service reimbursement methodologies issue payments to healthcare providers on the basis of the charges assigned to each of the separate services that were performed for the patient. Chargemasters are used to list the individual charges for every element entailed in providing a service (for example, surgical supplies, surgical equipment, room and board, nursing care, respiratory therapy, pharmaceuticals, medical equipment, and so on) (Casto and Layman 2011, 7–8).

107. **b** Charisma refers to influence by force of personality in which the leader inspires commitment, loyalty, and faith in a vision. Examples of people who have wielded such power include Winston Churchill, Martin Luther King, Jr., Michael Dell, and Barack Obama. Although the rhetoric and imagery can be stimulating to followers, there is a risk that with the leader's passing, leadership succession may fail and progress may falter (LaTour and Eichenwald Maki 2010, 659).

108. **a** Kouzes and Posner stressed that the relationship between leaders and followers has a synergy, in which the combination of their efforts produces more than either acting alone. This enthusiasm for change is essential in dealing more effectively with the innovations and changes that face modern organizations (LaTour and Eichenwald Maki 2010, 659).

109. **a** Quality standards (also known as service standards) are generally used by managers to monitor the performance quality of an individual employee, a functional unit, or the department as a whole. In this case, timely response to release of information requests can indirectly impact patient care. To properly communicate performance standards, managers need to make the distinction between quantitative and qualitative standards and identify examples of each for the HIS functions (LaTour and Eichenwald Maki 2010, 690).

110. **b** The average turnaround time was calculated by dividing the total response days attributed to the volume of routine requests that were responded to within the reporting period by the volume of routine requests responded to. $(200 \times 3) + (100 \times 5) + (50 \times 8) + (50 \times 10) / 400 = 5$ days (LaTour and Eichenwald Maki 2010, 697–698).

111. **c** Temporary variances are generally self-limiting. Temporary budget variances are not expected to continue in subsequent months (LaTour and Eichenwald Maki 2010, 799).

112. **a** For some transactions, such as the purchase of equipment or investment in marketable securities, there may be a change in the actual or perceived value of the underlying asset or liability. In those cases, adjustments or disclosures are made when reporting the financial data. Therefore, notes or disclosures that help the user make informed decisions must accompany all financial reports (LaTour and Eichenwald Maki 2010, 774–775).

113. **b** For financial reporting purposes, a fiscal year is divided into quarters (three-month periods) and months. Because the months generally end on the last calendar day, the quarters can be of slightly different duration. For example, the first quarter of a fiscal year that begins April 1 includes April, May, and June: 91 days. The second quarter of that same fiscal year includes July, August, and September: 92 days (LaTour and Eichenwald Maki 2010, 774).

114. **d** Although each step can require other steps and are not always done in the same order, virtually every financial transaction consists of these three fundamental steps: goods and services are provided, a transaction is recorded, and compensation is exchanged (LaTour and Eichenwald Maki 2010, 777).

115. **c** Accounts payable is a liability that is created when the organization has received goods or services but has not yet remitted the compensation. When the recipient of the goods and services does not intend to pay immediately, the amount is recorded by the recipient as an account payable. The recipient also records either the acquisition of an asset or the recognition of an expense (LaTour and Eichenwald Maki 2010, 779–780).

116. **c** The current ratio compares total current assets with total current liabilities:

$$\frac{4,000,000}{5,000,000} = \frac{4}{5} = 0.8$$

Total current assets / Total current liabilities

From this information, one can take the current assets (cash + accounts receivable + inventory) / current liabilities (accounts payable) = current ratio. The current ratio indicates that for every dollar of current liability, $0.80 of current assets could be used to discharge the liability, which is not enough because it is not at least $1 (LaTour and Eichenwald Maki 2010, 789).

117. **b** The difference between the budgeted fees and actual fees is an unfavorable variance of $2,000. Unfavorable variances occur when the actual results are worse than what was budgeted (LaTour and Eichenwald Maki 2010, 799).

118. **c** A simple method of capital project analysis is the accounting rate of return. This method compares the projected annual cash inflows, minus any applicable annual depreciation, divided by the initial investment. Consider the purchase of a CT scanner. Reimbursement from use of the machine is the cash inflow. Depreciation is easily calculated based on the initial investment (LaTour and Eichenwald Maki 2010, 803).

119. **c** ROI is most frequently used to analyze marketable securities retrospectively. The increase in market value of the securities divided by the initial investment is the ROI. Thus: $650,000 / $200,000 × 100 = 325% (LaTour and Eichenwald Maki 2010, 804).

120. **d** In this case, a profitability index helps the organization prioritize investment opportunities. For each investment, divide the present value of the cash inflows by the present value of the cash outflows (LaTour and Eichenwald Maki 2010, 804).

	Radiology	Cardiology	Pharmacy
Present value of cash inflows	$2,000,000	$1,200,000	$40,000
Present value of cash outflows	$500,000	$300,000	$10,000
Profitability Index	4	4	4

121. **a** The money that is in the payroll budget may not be spent by the end of the fiscal year; therefore, it is permanent. The payroll budget is the positive amount, so it is favorable (LaTour and Eichenwald Maki 2010, 799).

122. **b** It is unfavorable and permanent because money that was not in the budget was spent on consulting services (LaTour and Eichenwald Maki 2010, 799).

123. **c** When the operating budget has been developed and approved, it is the responsibility of the department management to ensure the budget goals are met (LaTour and Eichenwald Maki 2010, 799).

124. **d** Five major sources of accounting and reporting rules apply to healthcare organizations: the Financial Accounting Standards Board (FASB), the Securities and Exchange Commission (SEC), the Centers for Medicare and Medicaid Services (CMS), the Public Company Accounting Oversight Board (PCAOB), and the Internal Revenue Service (IRS). The SEC and PCAOB rules would not apply to this organization because they are a private organization (LaTour and Eichenwald Maki 2010, 775).

125. **c** The payback period is the time required to recoup the cost of an investment. Mortgage refinancing analysis frequently uses the concept of payback period. Mortgage refinancing is considered when interest rates have dropped. Refinancing may require upfront interest payments, called points, as well as a variety of administrative costs. In this example, the payback period is the time it takes for the savings in interest to equal the cost of the refinancing (LaTour and Eichenwald Maki 2010, 802).

126. **b** Partnerships survive as entities only so long as the partners remain together. A change in ownership dissolves the original partnership and a new one must be created (LaTour and Eichenwald Maki 2010, 776).

127. **a** The course of human history is marked with the contributions of great people. Such outstanding individuals originally led to the conception of leadership as an inborn ability, sometimes passed down through family, position, or social tradition, as in the cases of royal families in many parts of the world. The problem with the great person theory is that some of those who took positions of such greatness were terribly lacking (LaTour and Eichenwald Maki 2010, 651).

128. **d** Trait theory proposed that leaders possessed a collection of traits or personal qualities that distinguished them from nonleaders (LaTour and Eichenwald Maki 2010, 651–652).

129. **b** Internal change agents have the clear advantage of being familiar with the organization, its history, subtle dynamics, secrets, and resources. Such people are often well respected, securely positioned, and have the strong interpersonal relationships to foster change. There is an advantage to recognizing the internal expertise of employees, maintaining confidentiality of the process, and using people who are invested in the success of the outcome (LaTour and Eichenwald Maki 2010, 668).

130. **a** When asked about their early family and personal experiences, managers often describe uneventful early childhoods and see life as a steady normative progression of positive events and security. Being involved in social and organized activities from an early age, they tend to gain a strong sense of belonging, identity, and self-esteem from others. In contrast, leaders more often describe disruptive experiences in early family and childhood in which they were confronted by conflicts and stresses. These crises required reflection and mastery through which self-efficacy was developed. Because confidence grows out of problem solving rather than relationships, leaders may be more attached to a vision that drives their achievement and inspires others than to an immediate situation (Hickman 1990; Kempster 2006; Kotter 1990; Zaleznik 1977; LaTour and Eichenwald Maki 2010, 648).

131. **b** Telling stories about the future suggested by the trends has a number of advantages, including: most people are comfortable with this approach; findings are presented in an understandable and real-world context; stories are memorable, making it easier for others to remember essential points; and stories generate excitement and are fun to develop (LaTour and Eichenwald Maki 2010, 831).

132. **b** According to Tichy (1983), "the development of change strategy involves simultaneous attention to three [organizational] systems—technical, political, and cultural" (LaTour and Eichenwald Maki 2010, 836).

133. **d** Feedback controls are back-end processes that monitor and measure output, and then compare it to expectations and identify variations that then must be analyzed so correction action plans can be developed and implemented (LaTour and Eichenwald Maki 2010, 696).

134. **b** In reengineering, the entire manner and purpose of a work process is questioned. The goal is to achieve the desired process outcome in the most effective and efficient manner possible. Thus, the results expected from reengineering efforts include increased productivity, decreased costs, improved quality, maximized revenue, and more satisfied customers. However, it should be clearly understood that the main focus is on reducing costs (LaTour and Eichenwald Maki 2010, 707).

135. **c** Serial work division is the consecutive handling of tasks or products by individuals who perform a specific function in sequence. Often referred to as a production line work division, serial work division tends to create task specialists (LaTour and Eichenwald Maki 2010, 683).

136. **b** Changes to project scope are inevitable and should not be automatically considered a form of project failure. It is the way project changes are handled that can have a negative impact on the success of the project. The most important factor in scope change is for the stakeholders to understand the impact of the requested change and, if approved, be willing to accept the ramifications the change will have on the project's schedule and cost (LaTour and Eichenwald Maki 2010, 819).

137. **b**   A *Gantt chart* is used to illustrate project tasks, phases, and milestones, and their start, end, and completion dates. It helps to illustrate where more than one task must be performed simultaneously. The column labeled as B shows a check mark indicating the task "Load test data" is completed (Amatayakul 2012, 123–124).

138. **b**   Every project has an identified sponsor. The sponsor is the facility employee with the most vested interest in the project's success. It is a good practice to select someone who has responsibility for the organization's departments, divisions, and personnel that will be affected by the project (LaTour and Eichenwald Maki 2010, 808).

139. **b**   Assumptions are scope-limiting parameters. They provide constraints on what is and is not included in the project (LaTour and Eichenwald Maki 2010, 809).

140. **c**   The path with the greatest total duration time is called the critical path and represents the longest amount of time required to compete the total project. The critical path in this project is the sequence a → d → g → h → i, which will require 23 days (Shaw and Elliott 2012, 378).

141. **d**   A project manager supports the steering committee and is responsible for overseeing that all aspects of the EHR project are completed. A project manager requires skills much like a general contractor for a building project (Amatayakul 2012, 99).

142. **a**   In the project planning process, after all the tasks have been defined, the next step is to determine the dependency among tasks. The tasks in the project plan cannot all start at the same time. The definition of dependencies among the project tasks is the first step in scheduling the project. The purpose of the project schedule is to provide information on when the particular tasks can begin and when they are scheduled to end. In this situation, the tasks were not placed in priority order so that dependencies were not taken into account (LaTour and Eichenwald Maki 2010, 814).

143. **a**   To help all members understand the process, a team will undertake development of a flowchart. This work allows the team to thoroughly understand every step in the process and the sequence of steps. It provides a picture of each decision point and each event that must be completed. It readily points out places where there is redundancy and complex and problematic areas (LaTour and Eichenwald Maki 2010, 704).

144. **c**   A claim scrubber is used by facilities as an internal auditing system to limit the number of denied claims (Casto and Layman 2011, 252).

145. **a**   When a manager is planning to contract for staffing in a transitional situation in order to meet organizational goals, various types of arrangements can be considered; full-service contracting would be handing off a complete function to the contracted company (LaTour and Eichenwald Maki 2010, 687).

146. **b**   In-service education is a continuous process that builds on the basic skills learned through new employee orientation and on-the-job training. In-service education is concerned with teaching employees specific skills and behaviors required to maintain job performance or to retrain workers whose jobs have changed (LaTour and Eichenwald Maki, 748).

147. **b**   Implied consent is assumed when a patient voluntarily submits to medical treatment. The rationale behind this conclusion is that it is reasonable to assume the patients must understand the nature of the medical care or they would not submit to it (Odom-Wesley et al. 2009, 98).

148. **c**   When a state law is more stringent than a federal law, hospitals must comply with both (Odom-Wesley et al. 2009, 68).

149. **d**   Corporate negligence is a legal doctrine that was established by a judicial decision handed down in a 1965 court case, *Darling v. Charleston Community Hospital* (Odom-Wesley et al. 2009, 51).

150. **a**   Healthcare Integrity and Protection Data Bank was created to collect information on the legal actions (both civil and criminal) taken against licensed healthcare providers (Odom-Wesley et al. 2009, 52).

151. **d**   Privileged communication is a legal concept designed to protect the confidentiality between two parties (Brodnik et al. 2012, 5–6).

152. **c**   Privacy is the quality or state of being hidden from, or undisturbed by, the observation or activities of other persons or freedom from unauthorized intrusion; in healthcare-related contexts, the right of a patient to control disclosure of personal information (Brodnik et al. 2012, 5).

153. **c**   Competent adults have a general right to consent to or refuse medical treatment. If an adult has a sound mind or did when he or she created a living will, this patient has the right to refuse treatment (Brodnik et al. 2012, 149).

154. **b**   When obtaining consent for surgery, the surgeon is the healthcare provider who would discuss the consent for treatment with the patient. The basic elements of an informed surgical consent should include the purpose of the proposed procedure, any risks associated with the procedure, and if non-invasive treatment alternatives might be considered (Brodnik et al. 2012, 158).

155. **c**   Implied consent refers to consent for medical treatment that is communicated through some other means besides words. The patient communicates consent through his or her conduct: scheduling and arriving for the appointment and submitting to the exam or procedure without objection (Brodnik et al. 2012, 136).

156. **c**   The HIPAA Privacy Rule provides patients with significant rights that allow them to have some measure of control over their health information. As long as state laws or regulations or the physician does not state otherwise, competent adult patients have the right to access their health record (Brodnik et al. 2012, 218).

157. **c**   A facility may maintain a facility directory of patients being treated. HIPAA's Privacy Rule permits the facility to maintain in its directory the following information about an individual if the individual has not objected: name, location in the facility, and condition described in general terms. This information may be disclosed to persons who ask for the individual by name (Brodnik et al. 2012, 234).

158. **d**   HIM professionals must factor several criteria into their decision making. Ethicists provide assistance in this process. When faced with an ethical issue, the HIM professional should evaluate the ethical problem following these steps: determine the facts; consider the values and obligations of others; consider the choices that are both justified and not justified; identify prevention options. When a decision must be made about an issue and not identified following the steps, the decision most likely will be based on an individual's narrow moral perspective of right or wrong (LaTour and Eichenwald Maki 2010, 318).

159. **c** Section 164.528 of the Privacy Rule states that "an individual has the right to receive an accounting of disclosures made by a covered entity within the six years prior to the date on which the accounting is requested" (Brodnik et al. 2012, 243–244).

160. **c** Ownership of the health record is generally granted to the healthcare provider who generates the record. Since the record serves as both a medical document and as a legal document that provides proof of care, it is the "business" record of the healthcare provider (Brodnik et al. 2012, 329).

161. **c** Generally, if the patient is a minor at the time of treatment or hospitalization but has reached the age of majority at the time the authorization for access or disclosure of information is signed, the patient's authorization is legally required (Brodnik et al. 2012, 335).

162. **d** The Safe Medical Devices Act of 1990 was passed and then amended through the Medical Device Amendments of 1992. These Acts required facilities to report deaths and severe complications thought to be due to a device to the manufacturer and the Food and Drug Administration (FDA) through its MedWatch reporting system (LaTour and Eichenwald Maki 2010, 335).

163. **c** English common law is the primary source of many legal rules and principles and was based initially on tradition and custom. Common law, also known as judge-made law or case law, is regularly referred to as unwritten law originating from court decisions where no applicable statute exists (LaTour and Eichenwald Maki 2010, 272).

164. **b** Deidentified information is information from which personal characteristics have been removed and that, as a result, neither identifies nor provides a reasonable basis to believe it could identify an individual (Brodnik et al. 2012, 222).

165. **c** Treatment, payment, and healthcare operations (45 CFR 164.501) collectively referred to as TPO, are functions of a covered entity (CE) that are necessary for the CE to successfully conduct business. It is not the intent of the Privacy Rule to impose onerous rules that hinder a CE's functions. Thus, many of the Privacy Rule's requirements are relaxed or removed where PHI is needed for purposes of TPO (Brodnik et al. 2012, 226).

166. **c** The covered entity may require the individual to make an amendment request in writing and provide a rationale for it. Such a process must be communicated in advance to the individual through the organization's Notice of Privacy Practices. Therefore, an individual cannot review his or her physical record without an authorized HIM staff member present to maintain the integrity of the record (Brodnik et al. 2012, 242).

167. **b** For fundraising activities that benefit the covered entity (CE) (45 CFR 164.514 [f]) permits the CE to use or disclose to a business associate or an institutionally related foundation, without authorization, demographic information and dates of healthcare provided to an individual. The CE must inform individuals on its NPP that PHI may be used for this purpose. If a fundraising activity targets individuals based on their diagnosis, prior authorization is required (Brodnik et al. 2012, 248).

168. **c** The signature of the attending physician, next of kin, and insurance are not necessary on a HIPAA Complaint Authorization form. The Notice of Privacy Practices informs a patient how and when PHI can be released. If a particular use of information is not covered in the Notice of Privacy Practices, the patient must sign an authorization form specific to the additional disclosure before his or her information can be released (LaTour and Eichenwald Maki 2010, 194).

169. **b**   One of the most fundamental terms in the Privacy Rule is PHI, defined by the rule as "individually identifiable health information that is transmitted by electronic media, maintained in electronic media, or transmitted or maintained in any other form or medium" (45 CFR 160.103). To meet the individually identifiable element of PHI, information must meet all three portions of a three-part test. (1) It must either identify the person or provide a reasonable basis to believe the person could be identified from the information given. (2) It must relate to one's past, present, or future physical or mental health condition; the provision of healthcare; or payment for the provision of healthcare. (3) It must be held or transmitted by a covered entity or its business associate (Brodnik et al. 2012, 220–221).

170. **b**   The Joint Commission has established a cautious quality approach to the use of abbreviations in all its accredited organizations. To comply, every healthcare organization should strive to limit or eliminate the use of abbreviations by developing an organization-specific abbreviation list so that only those abbreviations approved by the organization are used. When more than one meaning for an approved abbreviation exists, an organization should choose only one meaning or context in which the abbreviation is to be used (Brodnik et al. 2012, 180–181).

171. **d**   The ruling handed down by a court to settle a dispute is called a judicial decision (Odom-Wesley et al. 2009, 281).

172. **b**   Because of the bioterrorism scares in recent years, the CDC is developing the National Electronic Disease Surveillance System (NEDSS), which serves as a major part of the Public Health Information Network (PHIN). It will provide a national surveillance system by connecting the CDC with local and state public health partners. This integrated system will allow the CDC to monitor trends from disease reporting at the local and state level to look for possible bioterrorism incidents (LaTour and Eichenwald Maki 2010, 339–340).

173. **b**   Every state has certain licensure regulations that healthcare facilities must meet in order to remain in operation. Licensure regulations may include very specific requirements for the content, format, retention, and use of patient records. These regulations are established by state governments, usually under the direction of state departments of health (LaTour and Eichenwald Maki 2010, 191).

174. **c**   The federal government Act that developed healthcare standards governing electronic data interchange and data security is the Health Insurance Portability and Accountability Act of 1996 (LaTour and Eichenwald Maki 2010, 177).

175. **b**   Most standards are created through a voluntary consensus process that involves identifying the need for a standard, negotiating the content of the standard, and drafting a proposed standard (LaTour and Eichenwald Maki 2010, 183).

176. **c**   Except in emergency situations, every surgical patient's chart must include a report of a complete history and physical conducted no more than seven days before the surgery is to be performed (Odom-Wesley et al. 2009, 150).

177. **a**   The Medicare reimbursement for long-term, acute-care hospitals (LTCHs) is under a PPS based on the Medicare MS-DRG system. The QIO is responsible for reviewing items such as medical necessity, reasonableness, and appropriateness of hospital admissions; inpatient hospital care for which outlier payments are sought; validity of the hospital's diagnostic and procedural information; completeness, adequacy, and quality of the services furnished in the hospital; and medical or other practices with respect to beneficiaries or billing for services furnished to the beneficiaries (Odom-Wesley et al. 2009, 351).

178. **c**   Core measures include Acute Myocardial Infarction (AMI), Heart Failure (HF), Pneumonia (PN), Surgical Care Improvement Project (SCIP), Pregnancy and Related Conditions (PR), Hospital Outpatient (HOP), Children's Asthma Care (CAC), and National Hospital Inpatient Quality Measures-Hospital-based Inpatient Psychiatric Services (HBIPS) (LaTour and Eichenwald Maki 2010, 537).

179. **c**   The formulary is composed of medications used for commonly occurring conditions/diagnosis treated in the healthcare organization. Organizations accredited by the Joint Commission are required to maintain a formulary and document that they review at least annually for a medication's continued safety and efficacy (Shaw and Elliott 2012, 212).

180. **b**   The development of the Patient Safety and Quality Improvement Act of 2005 and the National Patient Safety Goals have demonstrated that there is national focus on improving safety for patients (Shaw and Elliott 2012, 138).

Exam 2 Answers

1. **a**   The purpose of the Data Elements for Emergency Department Systems (DEEDS) is to support the uniform collection of data in hospital-based emergency departments and to substantially reduce incompatibilities in emergency department records. DEEDS recommends the collection of 156 data elements in hospitals that offer emergency care services. As with the UHDDS and UACDS, this data set contains recommendations on both the content and structure of the data elements to be collected (LaTour and Eichenwald Maki 2010, 169).

2. **c**   Health records and other documentation related to patient care are the property of the hospital or healthcare provider that created them (Odom-Wesley et al. 2009, 21).

3. **d**   The PASARR for MI/MR is required under the Omnibus Budget Reconciliation Act of 1987. It is completed preadmission and annually (Odom-Wesley et al. 2009, 369).

4. **d**   A line graph may be used to display time trends. The x-axis shows the unit of time from left to right, and the y-axis measures the values of the variable being plotted (LaTour and Eichenwald Maki 2010, 448).

5. **a**   The quality of coded clinical data depends on a number of factors, including validity. Validity is ensuring that the coded data is a correct representation of the patient's diagnosis and procedures (LaTour and Eichenwald Maki 2010, 399).

6. **d**   A consultation report is the documented findings and/or recommendation for further treatment by a physician or specialist. Consultations are usually performed at the request of the attending physician (Odom-Wesley et al. 2009, 354).

7. **d**   Data are the raw elements that make up our communications. Humans have the innate ability to combine data they collect and, through all their senses, produce information (which is data that have been combined to produce value), and enhance that information with experience and trial-and-error that produces knowledge (Amatayakul, 2012, 244).

8. **b**   The retention and destruction processes are subject to specific regulations in many states. Federal regulations and accreditation standards also include specific guidelines on the release and retention of patient-identified health information (Odom-Wesley et al. 2009, 23).

9. **b** Only when copies of the PHR are used for treatment can they be considered part of the facilities' legal health record (Odom-Wesley et al. 2009, 30).

10. **c** A longitudinal health record maintains information throughout the lifespan of the patient, ideally from birth to death (Amatayakul 2012, 12).

11. **d** One disadvantage of paper-based health records is the inability of an access control mechanism (Odom-Wesley et al. 2009, 217).

12. **d** An interval may be used for the patient's history and physical when the patient is readmitted within 30 days of the initial treatment for the same condition (Odom-Wesley et al. 2009, 108).

13. **c** The principal procedure is the procedure that was performed for the definitive treatment (rather than the diagnosis) of the main condition or a complication of the condition (LaTour and Eichenwald Maki 2010, 167).

14. **a** The attending physician principally responsible for the patient's hospital care writes and signs the discharge summary (Odom-Wesley et al. 2009, 200).

15. **b** A pathology report is a document that contains the diagnosis determined by examining cells and tissues under a microscope. The report may also contain information about the size, shape, and appearance of a specimen as it looks to the naked eye. This information is known as the gross description (Odom-Wesley et al. 2009, 171).

16. **c** In the past, the term "subacute care" was used in reference to the services provided to hospitalized patients who did not meet the medical criteria for needing acute care. Today, it refers to the level of skilled care needed by patients with complex medical conditions, typically Medicare patients who have multiple medical problems (LaTour and Eichenwald Maki 2010, 33).

17. **a** Main term: Depression, subterm: recurrent (Schraffenberger 2012, 29).

18. **c** Main term for procedure: Esophagoscopy, subterm: with closed biopsy. Code 45.16 is not correct because the endoscopy was advanced to the level of the esophagus and not to the level of the duodenum (Schraffenberger 2012, 41).

19. **d** Codes for symptoms, signs, and ill-defined conditions are not to be used as the principal diagnosis when a related definitive diagnosis has been established. The flank pain would not be coded because it is a symptom of the calculus (Schraffenberger 2012, 338–339).

20. **c** Main term for diagnosis: Incontinence, subterm: stress. Main term for procedure: Suspension, subterm: urethra (Schraffenberger 2012, 29).

21. **c** Begin with the main term of hernia repair; inguinal; incarcerated. The age of the patient and the fact that the hernia is not recurrent make the choice 49507 (Kuehn 2012, 20, 27, 164–165).

22. **c** Begin with the main term of Hernia repair; incisional. The fact that the hernia is recurrent, done via a laparoscope and is reducible make the choice 49656. Notice that the use of mesh is included in the code (Kuehn 2012, 20, 27, 164–165).

23. **b** Main term: Hysteroscopy; lysis; adhesions (Kuehn 2012, 20, 27).

24. **d** In the abdomen, peritoneum, and omentum subsection, the exploratory laparotomy is a separate procedure and should not be reported when it is part of a larger procedure. The code of 49000 is often used incorrectly because laparotomy is the approach to many abdominal surgeries. The code 58720 includes bilateral and so the –50 modifier is not necessary (Kuehn 2012, 156).

25. **c** Reliability is a measure of consistency of data items based on their reproducibility and an estimation of their error of measurement (LaTour and Eichenwald Maki 2010, 343).

26. **b** Hard coding is a term used in regard to the Chargemaster CPT codes that are automatically entered (Casto and Layman 2011, 250).

27. **c** Aging of accounts is maintained in 30-day increments (0–30 days, 31–60 days, and so forth) (Casto and Layman 2011, 253).

28. **c** Once the claim is submitted to the third-party payer for reimbursement, the accounts receivable clock begins to tick (Casto and Layman 2011, 253).

29. **b** Medicare Part B insurance covers physician services, medical services, and medical supplies not covered by Part A (durable medical equipment, mental healthcare, occupational, physical, and speech therapy, clinical laboratory services, and home health). It should be noted that the following healthcare services are usually not covered by Medicare Part A or B and are only covered by private health plans under the Medicare Advantage program: long-term nursing care, custodial care, dentures and dental care, eyeglasses, and hearing aids (LaTour and Eichenwald 2010, 376–377).

30. **d** Revenue cycle management is the supervision of all administrative and clinical functions that contribute to the capture, management, and collection of patient service revenue (Casto and Layman 2011, 249).

31. **b** The Department of Veterans Affairs provides covered healthcare services and supplies to eligible beneficiaries through the Civilian Health and Medical Program of the Department of Veterans Affairs (CHAMPVA) (Casto and Layman 2011, 89).

32. **d** A claim lists the fees or charges for each service (Casto and Layman 2011, 7).

33. **b** Nonparticipating providers (nonPARs) do not sign a participation agreement with Medicare but may or may not accept assignment. If the nonPAR physician elects to accept assignment, he or she is paid 95 percent (5 percent less than participating physicians) of the Medicare Fee Schedule (MFS). For example, if the MFS amount is $200, the PAR provider receives $160 (80 percent of $200), but the nonPAR provider receives only $152 (95 percent of $160). In this case, the physician is participating so he or she will receive 80 percent of the MFS or 80 percent of 300 = $240 (LaTour and Eichenwald Maki 2010, 405, 407).

34. **a** Because of the risks associated with miscommunication, verbal orders are strongly discouraged. To reduce miscommunication, the person receiving the order should read it back to ensure the order is correct. Verbal orders should be authenticated as soon as possible after they are given (Brodnik et al. 2012, 172).

35. **a** In 1997, the Joint Commission introduced the ORYX initiative to integrate outcomes data and other performance measurement data into its accreditation processes (LaTour and Eichenwald Maki 2010, 170).

36. **a** Data quality management functions involve continuous improvement for data quality throughout an organization and include four key processes for data. These processes are application, collection, warehousing, and analysis. Analysis is the process of translating data into information utilized for an application (Odom-Wesley et al. 2009, 385).

37. **a** The normal distribution is actually a theoretical family of distributions that may have any mean or any standard deviation. It is bell-shaped and symmetrical about the mean. Because it is symmetrical, 50 percent of the observations fall above the mean and 50 percent fall below it. In a normal distribution, the mean, median, and mode are equal (LaTour and Eichenwald Maki 2010, 457).

38. **c** A line graph is used to display time trends. The *x*-axis shows the unit of time from left to right, and the *y*-axis measures the number of prostate cancer deaths (LaTour and Eichenwald Maki 2010, 448).

39. **c** Data are the raw elements that make up our communications. Humans have the innate ability to combine data they collect and, through all their senses, produce information (which is data that have been combined to produce value), and enhance that information with experience and trial-and-error that produces knowledge (Amatayakul 2012, 244).

40. **a** These data are showing that Doctor X bills code 99213 primarily and not the other four service codes for established patients. However, the graph tells the reader nothing about Doctor X's documentation which would make answers b and c incorrect. Doctor X does use 99212 less than his peers, not more than his peers. A physician who consistently reports the same level of service for all patient encounters may look suspicious to claims auditors. With the exception of certain specialists, physicians treat all types of patients in their offices, and office treatment requires use of most of the levels of services (Kuehn 2012, 45).

41. **d** In this situation there are too many changes occurring at the same time to determine what is improving the nursing staffing satisfaction scores. Any one item could be the reason for the improvement. To evaluate the impact of the EHR nursing documentation component, a benefits realization study should have been utilized. This would have studied the impact of the EHR component before and after implementation (Amatayakul 2012, 137).

42. **b** The patient meets severity of illness with the persistent fever and intensity of service with the inpatient-approved surgery scheduled within 24 hours of admission (Shaw and Elliott 2012, 113, 120).

43. **b** The data shows that Dr. Jones' outcomes are all higher than the OB/GYN group. This data indicates that Dr. Jones should be monitored for continued poor performance compared to his peer group (Shaw and Elliott 2012, 298–301).

44. **a** The graph shows that the Asian population has increased in the last five years, so the organization may need to adjust staffing, offer a wider variety in dietary choices, and ensure patient rights and safety are appropriate in the face of possible language barriers, and religious and cultural differences (Shaw and Elliott 2012, 63–64).

45. **d** A gross autopsy rate is the proportion or percentage of deaths that are followed by the performance of autopsy. Using this data, five patients had autopsies performed out of the 25 deaths: 5 / 25 = 0.2 × 100 = 20% (LaTour and Eichenwald Maki 2010, 433).

46. **c**   Granting clinical privileges refers to the authorizing of a practitioner to provide specific patient care services within well-defined limits. The criteria for awarding clinical privileges must be detailed in the medical staff bylaws/rules and regulations (LaTour and Eichenwald Maki 2010, 543).

47. **d**   Discharge planning occurs during the patient's hospitalization and is conducted by a case manager or social worker in conjunction with the attending physician, patient, and patient's family and/or significant others. This planning process involves an assessment of the care level that the patient will need upon discharge from the current care setting. It may involve the placement of a patient in a skilled nursing facility or home care (Shaw and Elliott 2012, 113, 115).

48. **c**   Risk management systems today are sophisticated programs that function to identify, reduce, or eliminate potentially compensable events (PCEs), thereby decreasing the financial liability of injuries or accidents to patients, staff, or visitors (LaTour and Eichenwald Maki 2010, 549).

49. **c**   Finding ways to increase the rate of effective practice as applied to actual patient care are being analyzed. Many reasons for the gaps between best, evidence-based practice and current treatment choices include a gap in the dissemination of knowledge from research to practitioners; failure to implement best practice due to skepticism surrounding the cost effectiveness, environment, or organizational culture of practice setting; and research setting effectiveness not equating to an individual's practice setting (LaTour and Eichenwald Maki 2010, 519).

50. **b**   The National Association of Healthcare Quality (NAHQ) promotes continuous QI efforts in healthcare organizations by certifying qualified professionals. This organization offers QI professionals educational opportunities regardless of the healthcare setting they work in (LaTour and Eichenwald Maki 2010, 523).

51. **b**   As a method of improving the quality of care, outcomes management looks for the best treatment process. A treatment process is determined and used, and then data are collected and entered into a database. The data are analyzed and the treatment process altered as necessary. The goal is to find the best treatment possible to benefit patient care. These identified best practices can be considered guidelines to help clinicians make the best decisions possible for their patients. Outcomes research has changed clinical practice. Being able to collect meaningful data, and then analyze the types of treatments and the resulting outcomes, clinicians are able to provide better patient care more uniformly. Core measures, statement of outcomes, and clinical practice guidelines are all names of tools that can be used to measure the performance of an organization (LaTour and Eichenwald Maki 2010, 524–525).

52. **b**   Within both the quantitative and the qualitative approaches, researchers use inductive reasoning and deductive reasoning. Inductive reasoning, or induction, involves drawing conclusions based on a limited number of observations (LaTour and Eichenwald Maki 2010, 465).

53. **d**   Researchers use convenience samples when they "conveniently" use any unit that is at hand. For example, HIM professionals investigating physician satisfaction with departmental services could interview physicians who came to the department (LaTour and Eichenwald Maki 2010, 490).

54. **c**   The gross death rate is the proportion of all hospital discharges that ended in death. It is the basic indicator of mortality in a healthcare facility. The gross death rate is calculated by dividing the total number of deaths occurring in a given time period by the total number of discharges, including deaths, for the same time period: $25/500 = 0.05 \times 100 = 5\%$ (LaTour and Eichenwald Maki 2010, 431).

55. **b**   Epidemiological data are used to describe health-related issues or events, such as disease trends found in specific populations or general analytics of population health. The information then may be used to inform the public or generate actions that could affect a trend (LaTour and Eichenwald Maki 2010, 89).

56. **c**   The mode is the simplest measure of central tendency. It is used to indicate the most frequent observation in a frequency distribution. In this data set there are three occurrences of the value 8, and only two or less occurrences of any other value, so, 8 is the mode (LaTour and Eichenwald Maki 2010, 456).

57. **d**   An RFP generally includes the following: instructions for vendors; organizational objectives; background information of the organization; system goals and requirements; vendor qualifications; proposed solution; criteria to be used in evaluating the RFP; general contractual requirements; and pricing and support (LaTour and Eichenwald Maki 2010, 149–150).

58. **c**   To begin the planning process, the IS Steering Committee should review the organization's current strategic plans, goals, and objectives and evaluate its current external environment. The overall strategic plan should include an environmental assessment that analyzes the external forces that may affect the organization. External forces include changes in reimbursement methodologies, new government regulations, and changes in the demographics or healthcare needs of the community (LaTour and Eichenwald Maki 2010, 146).

59. **c**   Systems analysis is generally the first step in the systems development life cycle after the decision to implement the system has been made. It helps determine the needs for data, storage, reporting, and functionality (Sayles and Trawick 2010, 118).

60. **c**   In the analysis phase it is important to examine the current system and to identify opportunities for improvement or enhancement. Typically the existing system is evaluated by asking routine users to identify the strengths and limitations. Completion of this task can help ensure that the organization does not make a significant investment in a new system only to later discover what was needed was better communication, training, and more extensive technical support and not a new information system (LaTour and Eichenwald Maki 2010, 149).

61. **c**   Formal and informal mechanisms should be used to evaluate each vendor and its products. For example, the project team may hold vendor presentations, check references, attend user group meetings, and make site visits to other facilities that use the product. The purpose of these activities is to gather as much relevant information as possible to make an informed decision (LaTour and Eichenwald Maki 2010, 150).

62. **d**   The use case or script scenario is based on the organization's redesigned processes and asks the vendor how its products would perform the inherent functions. The approach is useful for avoiding yes and no responses (Amatayakul 2012, 386).

63. **c**   The Federated—inconsistent databases—model for HIE includes multiple enterprises agreeing to connect and share specific information in a point-to-point manner (Amatayakul 2012, 592–593).

64. **d**   A basic service provided by an HIE organization must be the actual transmission of the data. This is the technical networking service that provides appropriate bandwidth, latency, availability, ubiquity, and security (Amatayakul 2012, 597).

65. **d** An entity becomes a table in your relational database because it is the person, place, or thing about which you are collecting the data in your database. You would need to be able to query data on each entity from the database (Sayles and Trawick 2010, 96).

66. **d** A one-to-one relationship exists when an instance of an entity (a row or record) is associated with one instance of another entity, and vice versa. There is only one bed per patient and one patient per bed. One-to-one relationships are rare in logical-level data models because they often indicate a separate entity is unnecessary (Sayles and Trawick 2010, 96).

67. **b** Information capture is "the process of recording representations of human thought, perceptions, or actions in documenting patient care, as well as device-generated information that is gathered and/or computed about a patient as part of healthcare" (MRI 2002, 2). Some means of information capture in healthcare organizations are handwriting, speaking, word processing, touching a screen, pointing and clicking on words or phrases, videotaping, audio recording, and generating digital images through x-rays and scans (LaTour and Eichenwald Maki 2010, 117).

68. **b** The primary key (PK) for PATIENT, PATIENT_MRN, is repeated in VISIT, as is the PK for CLINIC, CLINIC_ID. These keys are called foreign keys (FK) in the VISIT table. Foreign keys allow relationships between tables. By having the foreign keys in VISIT, the information in PATIENT and CLINIC is linked through the VISIT table (LaTour and Eichenwald Maki 2010, 129).

69. **a** This model shows that the relationship between the data table (or entity) HOSPITAL and the data table (or entity) DIVISION is one-to-many. A one-to-many relationship means that for every instance of HOSPITAL stored in the database, many related instances of DIVISION may be stored. Reading the diagram in the other direction, each instance of DIVISION stored in the database is related to only one instance of HOSPITAL (Sayles and Trawick 2010, 96).

70. **a** Extranets are networks that connect a given organization to its customers and business partners or suppliers (business associates in healthcare). Although extranets send information over public networks, requiring a greater level of security, access to them is still restricted to the services and persons authorized (Amatayakul 2012, 300).

71. **c** A data warehouse is a database that has the following functions: serves as a neutral storage area for data extracted from an organization's transactional systems, serves as a storage area organized around specific business functions or requirements, and provides easy access to business data for analysis or data mining (that is, decision support) (LaTour and Eichenwald Maki 2010, 608).

72. **b** A database is a term used to refer to an organized collection of data that have been stored electronically to facilitate easy access (Odom-Wesley et al. 2009, 224).

73. **b** Terminal digit filing is a common method of paper record filing. Records are filed according to a three-part number made up of two-digit pairs (LaTour and Eichenwald Maki 2010, 218–219).

74. **c** Clinical decision support systems help physicians and other clinicians make diagnostic and treatment decisions within the electronic record (Odom-Wesley et al. 2009, 231).

75. **c** Standardization of abbreviations helps ensure the quality and completeness of health record content in both paper-based and computer-based environments (Odom-Wesley et al. 2009, 227).

76. **b** In the centralized database model, all the organization's patient health information is stored in one system (Odom-Wesley et al. 2009, 225).

77. **a** Questionnaires allow for a large number of users to provide input about the needs of the system (Sayles and Trawick 2010, 119).

78. **a** An accession number consists of the first digits of the year the patient was first seen at the facility, with the remaining digits assigned sequentially throughout the year. The first case in, for example, might be 09-0001. The accession number may be assigned manually or by the automated cancer database used by the organization. An accession registry of all cases can be kept manually or be provided as a report by the database software (LaTour and Eichenwald Maki 2010, 332).

79. **d** Risk analysis is a systematic process of identifying security measures to afford protections given an organization's specific environment, including where the measures are located, what level of automation they have, how sensitive the information is that needs protection, what remediation will cost, and many other factors (LaTour and Eichenwald Maki 2010, 252).

80. **c** Master population/patient index (MPI) contains patient-identifiable data such as name, address, date of birth, dates of hospitalizations or encounters, name of attending physician, and health record number (LaTour and Eichenwald Maki 2010, 331).

81. **b** As within any type of setting, the most common security threat to a health information system is an internal threat within the organization by employees (Brodnik et al. 2012, 296–297).

82. **c** Context-based access is the most stringent type of access control. It takes into account the person attempting to access the data, the type of data being accessed, and the context of the transaction in which the access attempt is made (Brodnik et al. 2012, 304).

83. **b** Authenticity is the verification of a record's validity. It confirms that it is the record of the individual in question and it is what it purports to be, and therefore, its reliability and truthfulness as evidence (Brodnik et al. 2012, 174).

84. **c** Contingency or disaster recovery planning (DRP) is an important component of protecting ePHI. Healthcare providers need plans in the event of a power failure, disaster, or other emergency that limits or eliminates access to facilities and ePHI (Brodnik et al. 2012, 318–319).

85. **b** The recognition of constrained or unconstrained, handwritten, English language free text (print or cursive, upper- or lowercase, characters or symbols) typically stored on paper-based, analog documents is known as intelligent character recognition (ICR) technology (LaTour and Eichenwald Maki 2010, 55).

86. **a** Data repositories in healthcare organizations require tools designed to perform intricate data searches and retrievals using online/real-time transaction processing (OLTP) (LaTour and Eichenwald Maki 2010, 58).

87. **b** Diagnostic image data, such as a digital chest x-ray or a computed tomography (CT) scan stored in a diagnostic image management system, represent a different type of data called bit-mapped data. The format of bit-mapped data also is unstructured. Saving each bit of the original image creates the image file (LaTour and Eichenwald Maki 2010, 52).

88. **a** The bar code symbol was standardized for the healthcare industry making it easier to adopt bar-coding technology. Bar-coding applications have been adopted for labels, patient wristbands, specimen containers, business/employee/patient records, library reference materials, medication packages, dietary items, paper documents, and more (LaTour and Eichenwald Maki 2010, 55).

89. **a** Fuzzy logic is a rules-based system that mimics human thought and enables a computer to "think" in inexact terms rather than in a definitive, either-or manner. Expert systems "learn" based on the continual addition of data to the system (Sayles and Trawick 2010, 101).

90. **a** Autoauthentication is a policy that allows the physician or provider to state in advance that dictated and transcribed reports should automatically be considered approved and signed when the physician does not make corrections within a certain period of time. Another variation of autoauthentication is that physicians authorize the HIM department to send a weekly list of documents needing signatures. The list is then signed and returned to the HIM department (LaTour and Eichenwald Maki 2010, 213).

91. **c** Physiological signal processing systems measure biological signals (for example, ECG, EEG, EMG, and fetal trace systems). They help to integrate the medical science of analyzing the signals with such disciplines as biomedical engineering, computer graphics, mathematics, diagnostic image processing, computer vision, and pattern recognition (LaTour and Eichenwald Maki 2010, 69).

92. **d** The MPI includes data elements necessary to identify a patient. These elements include date of birth, complete address, phone numbers, health record number, billing or account number, name of attending physician, dates of admission and discharge, disposition, marital status, gender, race, and patient's emergency contact (LaTour Eichenwald Maki 2010, 226).

93. **b** Employee assistance programs are a type of behavioral healthcare setting in which employees are given access to psychological counseling on a limited basis (Odom-Wesley et al. 2009, 433).

94. **c** The discipline of ergonomics has helped redefine the employee workspace with consideration for comfort and safety (LaTour and Eichenwald Maki 2010, 682).

95. **a** The rectangle symbol in a flowchart is called a process icon and represents periods in the process when actions are being performed by human participants (Shaw and Elliott 2012, 166).

96. **d** First calculate the number of productive hours in a day: 88% × 8 hours = 7.04 hours/day. Then determine the number of charts filed per record filer: 1,000 / 3 = 333.3. Then divide 333 charts / 7 hours = 47.5 or 48 charts/hour per productive FTE (LaTour and Eichenwald Maki 2010, 690).

97. **b** Organization is the planned coordination of the activities of more than one person for the achievement of a common purpose or goal. It is accomplished through the division of labor, and it is based on a hierarchy of authority and responsibility. Jobs and the people who perform them are arranged in a way that accomplishes the goals of the organization (LaTour and Eichenwald Maki 2010, 718).

98. **c** The organizational chart shows the organization's various activities and the specific members or categories of members assigned to carry out its activities (LaTour and Eichenwald Maki 2010, 720).

99. **a** Quantity standards (also called productivity standards) and quality standards (also known as service standards) are generally used by managers to monitor individual employee performance and the performance of a functional unit or the department as a whole. To properly communicate performance standards, managers need to make the distinction between quantitative and qualitative standards and identify examples of each for the HIS functions (LaTour and Eichenwald Maki 2010, 690).

100. **b** Quantity standards (also called productivity standards) and quality standards (also known as service standards) are generally used by managers to monitor individual employee performance and the performance of a functional unit or the department as a whole. To properly communicate performance standards, managers need to make the distinction between quantitative and qualitative standards and identify examples of each for the HIS functions (LaTour and Eichenwald Maki 2010, 690).

101. **c** Performance counseling usually begins with informal counseling or a verbal warning. No record of these actions is maintained in the employee's file (LaTour and Eichenwald Maki 2010, 735).

102. **c** Conflict management focuses on working with the individuals involved to find a mutually acceptable solution. There are three ways to address conflict: compromise, control, and constructive confrontation (LaTour and Eichenwald Maki 2010, 736).

103. **a** The Hay method of job evaluation, officially known as the Hay Guide Chart-Profile Method of Job Evaluation, is widely used as a job evaluation tool (LaTour and Eichenwald Maki 2010, 735).

104. **c** A teleconferencing network usually consists of video and audio recording equipment and a satellite service to broadcast the signal to televisions in a remote location. Videoconferencing permits additional flexibility in delivering courses that may be enhanced through visual as well as audio presentation, such as those that include demonstrations or simulation exercises. It is useful for training employees in organizations with multiple sites, such as integrated delivery networks with inpatient and outpatient facilities. The expense is justified for large organizations that do extensive training (LaTour and Eichenwald Maki 2010, 757).

105. **a** Delegation is the process of distributing work duties and decision making to others. To be effective, delegation should be commensurate with authority and responsibility. A manager must assign responsibility, which is an expectation that another person will perform tasks. At the same time, authority, or the right to act in ways necessary to carry out assigned tasks, must be granted (LaTour and Eichenwald Maki 2010, 763).

106. **b** One of the significant consequences of the organization and its leaders not being perceived as highly ethical is that employees feel less loyalty and commitment and tend to leave the organization (LaTour and Eichenwald Maki 2010, 659–660).

107. **d** In what has become a classic case, the 1987 *Price-Waterhouse v. Hopkins* case reflected the prominent role of gender stereotype. Ann Hopkins was a high-performing and rapidly rising employee who during five years had brought in more clients than other candidates for company partnership. When she was denied partnership status, she sued. Allegedly, partners at what was then Price-Waterhouse perceived her direct and assertive behavior as inappropriate for what they believed should be a feminine role. They told her she was "too macho, abrasive, and overbearing" and would be more promotable if she wore jewelry and makeup and walked and talked more femininely (*Price-Waterhouse* 1987). Price-Waterhouse was cited for sex discrimination, and the impact of gender stereotypes on people and organizations was brought to prominence (LaTour and Eichenwald Maki 2010, 661).

108. **a** Reductionism occurs when complex processes are reduced to their constituent elements and analyzed by their parts (LaTour and Eichenwald Maki 2010, 662).

109. **c** Employees work full- or part-time in their own homes. The first employees in HIS departments to take advantage of telecommuting were transcriptionists; they were soon followed by at-home coders. These telecommuters use computers (often provided by the facility) at home to transcribe or code information and then transmit it electronically back to the HIS department (LaTour and Eichenwald Maki 2010, 686).

110. **c** When an organization has delivered goods and/or services, payment for same is expected. Because the revenue has been accrued upon delivery or provision of the goods and services, the organization must have some way to keep track of what is owed to them as a result. Accounts receivable then is merely a list of the amounts due from various customers (in this case, patients). Payment on the individual amounts is expected within a specified period. A schedule of those expected amounts is prepared in order to track and follow up on payments that are overdue (late) (LaTour and Eichenwald Maki 2010, 793–794).

111. **a** Along with the recording of clinical documentation is the capture of the associated billing information. Regardless of the reimbursement system, the organization must capture the billable event in such a way that the financial transaction can be completed. Therefore, when a medication is administered to a patient, the clinical record reflects the medication, dosage, time, date, and route of administration, and the clinical personnel who administered it. At the same time, the charge for the drug must be communicated to patient accounts. This detailed tracking of billable events also supports the cost accounting function (LaTour and Eichenwald Maki 2010, 777–778).

112. **b** The net income is based only on the arithmetic difference between total revenue and total expenses of the current fiscal year. The difference between the total revenue of $2,500,000 and the total expenses of $2,250,000 is $250,000 (LaTour and Eichenwald Maki 2010, 785).

113. **d** In a not-for-profit environment, the difference between assets and liabilities is referred to as the fund balance or just net assets. These relationships can be expressed in the following equation:

$$\text{Assets} - \text{Liabilities} = \text{Net assets (equity)}$$

In this example, add the assets (cash, A/R, building and land, which is $2,450,000) and then subtract the liabilities (A/P and mortgage which is $950,000) or $1,700,000 (LaTour and Eichenwald Maki 2010, 781).

114. **d** In a not-for-profit environment, the difference between assets and liabilities is referred to as the fund balance or just net assets. These relationships can be expressed in the following equation:

$$\text{Assets} - \text{Liabilities} = \text{Net assets (equity)}$$

In this example, add the assets (cash, A/R, building and land, which is $2,450,000) and then subtract the liabilities (A/P and mortgage which is $950,000) or $1,700,000 + $250,000 of income or $1,950,000 (LaTour and Eichenwald Maki 2010, 781).

115. **b** Accumulated depreciation is an example of a contra-account (LaTour and Eichenwald Maki 2010, 779).

116. **d** Regardless of the purchasing system used, controls must be in place to ensure the efficient execution of approved transactions. Purchase orders, shipping/receiving documents, and invoices are the key controls over the purchase process (LaTour and Eichenwald Maki 2010, 782).

117. **d** The payback period is the time required to recoup the cost of an investment. Mortgage refinancing analysis frequently uses the concept of payback period. Mortgage refinancing is considered when interest rates have dropped. Refinancing may require up-front interest payments, called points, as well as a variety of administrative costs. In this example, the payback period is the time it takes for the savings in interest to equal the cost of the refinancing. For this problem, it is asking how long it will take to pay back the money spent to refinance. The hospital is spending $12,000 to refinance and will save $500 a month once they do. The payback period, or time to "recoup their costs," is 12,000/500 = 24. This is 24 months (LaTour and Eichenwald Maki 2010, 802).

118. **c** The disadvantage of a payback period is that it ignores the time value of money. Because the funds used for one capital investment could have been invested elsewhere, there is always an inherent opportunity cost of choosing one investment over another. Hence, there is an assumed rate of return against which investments are compared and a benchmark rate of return under which a facility will not consider an investment (LaTour and Eichenwald Maki 2010, 803).

119. **c** Materiality refers to the thresholds below which items are not considered significant for reporting purposes. These thresholds may be a dollar value or percentage of a dollar value (LaTour and Eichenwald Maki 2010, 774).

120. **c** 501(c)(3) organizations are largely exempt from federal taxes but must confine their activities to the public benefit. Donations to 501(c)(3) organizations are generally tax deductible (for the donor) to the extent that no goods or services have been received in return. For that reason, charities are generally 501(c)(3) organizations, and many 501(c)(6) organizations have charitable components that are separately incorporated. For example, AHIMA is a 501(c)(6) organization that has a 501(c)(3) component, the AHIMA Foundation (LaTour and Eichenwald Maki 2010, 776–777).

121. **c** Certain long-term assets, such as equipment and furniture, wear out over time and must be replaced. Such assets contribute to revenue over multiple fiscal periods. Therefore, the cost of these assets is not recorded as an expense at the time of purchase. Rather, the current asset, cash, is exchanged for a long-term asset, equipment. A portion of the historical cost of equipment then is moved from asset into expense each fiscal year and cumulated into the contra-account: accumulated depreciation. Eventually, the cost of equipment has been expensed and equipment account value is zero. The purpose of depreciation is to spread the cost of an asset over its useful life. The straight-line depreciation of this item is calculated by taking the cost of the item minus the residual value and dividing that by the useful life. 10,000 − 500/5 = $1,900 (LaTour and Eichenwald Maki 2010, 779).

122. **a** A balance sheet is a snapshot of the accounting equation at a point in time (LaTour and Eichenwald Maki 2010, 785–786).

123. **d** In a paper-based accounting system, journal entries are recorded chronologically in a general journal and their component debits and credits are posted to the individual accounts. The list of all the individual accounts is referred to as the general ledger. In a computer-based environment, only the original journal entry is posted. The computer stores the entries and generates summaries of the individual accounts on request (LaTour and Eichenwald Maki 2010, 784–785).

124. **c** The result of this completed transaction is an increase in cash and an increase in equity (revenue) (LaTour and Eichenwald Maki 2010, 784).

125. **b**   Zero-based budgets apply to organizations for which each budget cycle poses the opportunity to continue or discontinue services based on the availability of resources. Every department or activity must be justified and prioritized annually in order to effectively allocate the organization's resources. Professional associations and charitable foundations, for example, routinely use zero-based budgeting (LaTour and Eichenwald Maki 2010, 797).

126. **a**   The Vertical Dyad Linkage (VDL) represents micro theories that focus on dyadic relationships, or those between two people or between a leader and a small group. More specifically, they explain how in-group and out-group relationships form with a leader or mentor, and how delegation may occur (LaTour and Eichenwald Maki 2010, 656–657).

127. **d**   When the combination of leader effectiveness and gender is questioned, the answer becomes clearer, and middle managers who were described as successful more often possessed a combination of stereotypical masculine and feminine qualities or were androgynous leaders (Korabik 1990; LaTour and Eichenwald Maki 2010, 662).

128. **d**   Strategic management is a process a leader uses for assessing a changing environment to create a vision of the future, determining how the organization fits into the anticipated environment based on its mission, vision, and knowledge of its strengths, weaknesses, opportunities, and threats, and then setting in motion a plan of action to position the organization accordingly (LaTour and Eichenwald Maki 2010, 824).

129. **a**   Strategic management and thinking should be viewed as a component of each of the five functions of management. Every aspect of management involves a strategic management component (LaTour and Eichenwald Maki 2010, 825–826).

130. **a**   A vision statement conveys a picture of what the future will look like (LaTour and Eichenwald Maki 2010, 827).

131. **a**   Sound change strategies and tactics alone do not ensure success. Success depends on great execution, including securing support for the needed organizational change efforts (LaTour and Eichenwald Maki 2010, 836).

132. **a**   Parallel work division is the concurrent handling of tasks. Multiple employees do identical types of tasks and basically see the process through from beginning to end (LaTour and Eichenwald Maki 2010, 684).

133. **b**   Basic work distribution data can be collected in a work distribution chart, which is initially filled out by each employee and includes all responsible task content. Task content should come directly from the employee's current job description. In addition to task content, each employee tracks each task's start time, end time, and volume or productivity within a typical workweek. The results of a work distribution analysis can lead a department to redefine the job descriptions of some employees, redesign the office layout, or establish new or revised procedures for some department functions in order to gain improvements in staff productivity or service quality (LaTour and Eichenwald Maki 2010, 684).

134. **d**   Determining the work schedule for departmental staff involves more than simply assigning the correct number of work hours to each employee. Effective scheduling results in the following: core of employees on duty at all times when services must be provided; a pattern of hours (shifts) to be worked and days off that employees can be reasonably sure will not change except in extreme emergencies; and fair and just treatment of all employees with regard to hours assigned (LaTour and Eichenwald Maki 2010, 684–685).

135. **d**   A well-defined project has specific objectives. After the project's objectives have been defined, all project activities should be focused on meeting them. The project activities result in project deliverables or work products (LaTour and Eichenwald Maki 2010, 808).

136. **d**   One reason why many projects fail to meet their objectives within the expected time frame and budget is that their scope begins to grow as they progress. For example, new functions or features are added to a software implementation. This is commonly known as scope creep (LaTour and Eichenwald Maki 2010, 809).

137. **a**   A psychological risk would be a project that introduces a significant change to a department employee's responsibilities. The change positions the employee out of his or her comfort zone. Before the project begins, an employee may be considered an expert in his or her job responsibilities. At the conclusion of the project, the same employee may have new duties and will not have the same proficiency in them. This could cause self-esteem problems. It is common for employee turnover to occur during a project because of this threat to job security (LaTour and Eichenwald Maki 2010, 809).

138. **b**   An EHR steering committee or project sponsorship may go by different names; virtually every organization that undertakes an EHR project forms a steering committee of some type to initiate the project and gain representation from all stakeholders in product selection and implementation (Amatayakul 2012, 98).

139. **a**   The row numbers in the project plan identify each element in the plan (Amatayakul 2012, 121).

140. **c**   Releasing accurate information for public health purposes for patients with communicable diseases, such as AIDS or venereal disease, and assisting with the complexities of information management in the context of bioterrorism and the threat or reality of global diseases, such as smallpox or Avian flu, is an ethical responsibility of the HIM professional (LaTour and Eichenwald Maki 2010, 314).

141. **b**   If one thing can be accurately predicted about a project, it is that it will not progress as scheduled. To account for the inevitable changes, the project manager should perform a risk analysis and adjust the project schedule, work effort, or cost projections to incorporate any anticipated risk (LaTour and Eichenwald Maki 2010, 817).

142. **b**   HIM professionals must be aware of the retention statutes and retention periods in his or her state of employment and any federal statutes that apply. In some cases, the organization may define a retention period that is longer than the period required by the state. The organization should base its retention policy on hospital and medical needs and any applicable statutes and regulations (LaTour and Eichenwald Maki 2010, 282).

143. **a**   After the tasks have been defined, the project manager determines who will perform each task (resources), the amount of effort it will take to complete the task (work), and how long it will take to finish the task (duration). Work and duration are two different values (LaTour and Eichenwald Maki 2010, 815).

144. **b** Visually, transactions have two sides: left and right. Debits are shown on the left; credits are shown on the right. Each account has two sides: increase and decrease. In asset accounts, the left-hand debit side represents the natural balance of the account, and debits increase the account. Conversely, credits decrease an asset account. Obviously, for the accounting equation to balance, the opposite is true of liability and equity accounts. The right-hand credit side of liability and equity accounts represents the natural balance, and credits increase the accounts. Instead of using minus signs or brackets to represent the increases and decreases, debits and credits provide an additional safeguard against clerical error because every transaction must balance (LaTour and Eichenwald Maki 2010, 783).

145. **a** The acid-test ratio compares current liabilities to the current assets that are truly liquid, that is, able to be turned into cash quickly (LaTour and Eichenwald Maki 2010, 789).

146. **d** The base rate for failed leadership has been estimated between 65 percent and 75 percent—based on employees reporting that the worst aspect of their job is their immediate supervisor (Hogan and Kaiser, 2004; LaTour and Eichenwald Maki 2010, 648).

147. **d** A regulation is a rule established by an administrative agency of government (LaTour and Eichenwald Maki 2010, 273).

148. **d** Redisclosure is the process of releasing health record documentation originally created by a different provider (Odom-Wesley et al. 2009, 67).

149. **c** Retention policies dictate how long individual health records must remain available for authorized use (Odom-Wesley et al. 2009, 67).

150. **d** The distinction of psychotherapy notes is important due to HIPAA requirements that these notes may not be released unless specifically specified in an authorization (Odom-Wesley et al. 2009, 440).

151. **d** Refuse to participate in or conceal unethical practices or procedures. AHIMA professionals must abide to the AHIMA Code of Ethics (LaTour and Eichenwald Maki 2010, 310–311).

152. **d** When a person or entity that willfully and knowingly violates the HIPAA Privacy Rule with the intent to sell, transfer, or use PHI for commercial advantage, personal gain, or malicious harm, a fine of not more than $250,000, not more than 10 years in jail, or both may be imposed (LaTour and Eichenwald Maki 2010, 291).

153. **b** The basic elements of an informed consent should include the purpose of the proposed procedure, any risks associated with the procedure, and if any noninvasive treatment alternatives (Brodnik et al. 2012, 137).

154. **d** The Patient Self-Determination Act, which is part of the Omnibus Budget Reconciliation Act of 1990, requires healthcare providers to inform patients of their right to create advance directives, document the presence or absence of an advance directive in a patient's health record, and ensure compliance with state law respecting advance directives (Brodnik et al. 2012, 146–147).

155. **c** Competent adults have a general right to consent to or refuse medical treatment. If an adult has a sound mind or did when he or she created a living will, this patient has the right to refuse treatment (Brodnik et al. 2012, 149–150).

156. **b** By virtue of their age, minors are generally considered legally incompetent and unable to consent to their own treatment. Therefore, the consent of a parent or other legal guardian is required. If the minor's parents are divorced, only one parent needs to consent for treatment (Brodnik et al. 2012, 154-156).

157. **c** When obtaining consent for treatment, the physician is the healthcare provider who would discuss the treatment with the patient. The basic elements of an informed consent should include the purpose of the proposed procedure, any risks associated with the procedure, and if any noninvasive treatment alternatives (Brodnik et al. 2012, 137).

158. **c** Applicable statutes of limitations, the time period in which a lawsuit may be filed, must be considered in establishing a retention schedule (Brodnik et al. 2012, 188).

159. **c** The Privacy Rule introduced the standard that individuals should be informed of how covered entities use or disclose protected health information (PHI). This notice must be provided to an individual at his or her first contact with the covered entity (Brodnik et al. 2012, 227).

160. **a** There are circumstances in which PHI can be used or disclosed without the individual's written authorization and for which the individual does not have the opportunity to agree or object. These would include use and disclosure of medical information for treatment, payment, and operations (Brodnik et al. 2012, 235).

161. **c** The Privacy Rule's general requirement is that authorization must be obtained for uses and disclosure of protected health information (PHI) created for research that includes treatment of the individual (Brodnik et al. 2012, 237).

162. **c** The custodian of health records is the individual who has been designated as having responsibility for the care, custody, control, and proper safekeeping and disclosure of health records for such persons or institutions that prepare and maintain records of healthcare (Brodnik et al. 2012, 7–8).

163. **c** An outsourced transcription company and vendor would be business associates of a covered entity (CE). A business associate is a person or organization other than a member of a CE's workforce that performs functions or activities on behalf of or affecting a CE that involve the use or disclosure of individually identifiable health information (45 CFR 160.103[1]; Brodnik et al. 2012, 220).

164. **b** The Privacy Rule permits individuals to request that a covered entity amend PHI or a record about the individual in a designated record set. Because the incident report was erroneously placed in this patient's record, it is not part of the designated record set and not amendable by the patient (Brodnik et al. 2012, 407).

165. **b** The law firm of Hall and Hall is a business associate of Champion Hospital because it performs activities on behalf of the hospital and uses and discloses individually identifiable information. A business associate is a person or organization other than a member of a covered entity's workforce that performs functions or activities on behalf of or affecting a covered entity that involve the use or disclosure of individually identifiable health information (45 CFR 160.103(1); Brodnik et al. 2012, 220).

166. **b** The review of the medical record by a medical staff committee is approved use of protected health information (PHI). The Privacy Rule provides a broad list of activities that fall under the umbrella of healthcare operations including quality assessment and improvement and case management (Brodnik et al. 2012, 226).

167. **c** Covered entities are responsible for their workforce, which consists not only of employees but also volunteers, student interns, and trainees. Workforce members are not limited to those who receive wages from the CE (45 CFR 160.103; Brodnik et al. 2012, 219).

168. **b** Although a person or organization may, by definition, be subject to the Privacy Rule by virtue of the type of organization it is, not all information that it holds or comes into contact with is protected by the Privacy Rule. For example, the Privacy Rule has specifically excluded from its scope employment records held by the covered entity in its role as employer (45 CFR 160.103). Under this exclusion, employee physical examination reports contained within personnel files are specifically exempted from this rule (Brodnik et al. 2012, 226).

169. **c** A healthcare facility may maintain a facility directory of patients being treated. Once the individual has agreed, the Privacy Rule permits the facility to maintain in its directory the following information about an individual: name, location in its facility, condition described in general terms, and religious affiliation (Brodnik et al. 2012, 234).

170. **a** Accreditation is the act of granting approval to a healthcare organization. The approval is based on whether the organization has met a set of voluntary standards that were developed by the accreditation agency. The Joint Commission is an example of an accreditation agency (Shaw and Elliott 2012, 330).

171. **d** A discharge summary must be completed within 30 days after discharge for most patients but within 24 hours for patients transferred to other facilities. Discharge summaries are not always required for patients who were hospitalized for less than 48 hours (LaTour and Eichenwald Maki 2010, 200–201).

172. **a** The Patient Self-Determination Act (PSDA 1991) requires healthcare facilities to inform patients of their rights under state law to make advance decisions concerning medical care by activating advance directives (Odom-Wesley et al. 2009, 412–413).

173. **a** Abstracting is the function of compiling the pertinent information from the medical record based on predetermined data sets (LaTour and Eichenwald Maki 2010, 91).

174. **a** In peer review, a member of a profession assesses the work of colleagues within that same profession. Peer review has traditionally been at the center of quality assessment and assurance efforts. The medical profession's peer review efforts have emphasized the scientific aspects of quality. Appropriate use of pharmaceuticals, postoperative infection rates, and accuracy of diagnosis are among the measures of quality that have been used. Peer review is a requirement of both CMS and the Joint Commission (LaTour and Eichenwald Maki 2010, 34).

175. **c** Joint Commission, Commission on Accreditation of Rehabilitation Facilities, and the National Committee for Quality Assurance are all acceptable accrediting bodies for behavioral healthcare settings (Odom-Wesley et al. 2009, 447).

176. **b** The purpose of the identifier standards are to establish methods for assigning unique identifiers to individual patients, healthcare professionals, healthcare provider organizations, and healthcare vendors and suppliers (Odom-Wesley et al. 2009, 311).

177. **c**   State licensure agencies have regulations that are modeled after the Medicare Conditions of Participation and Joint commission standards. States conduct annual surveys to determine the hospital's continued compliance with licensure standards (Odom-Wesley et al. 2009, 287).

178. **b**   One of the five categories of health informatics standards is vocabulary standards. Its purpose is to establish uniform definitions for clinical terms (Odom-Wesley et al. 2009, 310).

179. **c**   The rule mandates that healthcare-covered entities and business partners implement a common standard (ASC X12N) for the transfer of information and accept the standard-based electronic transaction. This regulation does not apply to the transfer of data and information within a healthcare organization, but it does apply to the transfer of data and information external to and between healthcare organizations (LaTour and Eichenwald Maki 2010, 56–57).

180. **b**   Sometimes the patient's health status may make communication impossible, such as when a patient is incapacitated by a head injury or stroke. Through advance directives, the law provides a means for individuals to communicate their healthcare wishes in advance should they become incapacitated (Brodnik et al. 2012, 143).

References

RHIA

Primary References

Amatayukul, M.K. 2012. *Electronic Health Records: A Practical Guide for Professionals and Organizations,* 5th ed. Chicago: American Health Information Management Association.

Brodnik, M., L. Rinehart-Thompson, and R. Reynolds. 2012. *Fundamentals of Law for Health Informatics and Information Management,* 2nd Edition. Chicago: American Health Information Management Association.

Casto, A. and E. Layman. 2011. *Principles of Healthcare Reimbursement,* 3rd ed. Chicago: American Health Information Management Association.

Horton, L. 2012. *Calculating and Reporting Healthcare Statistics,* 4th ed. Chicago: American Health Information Management Association.

Kuehn, L. 2012. *Procedural Coding and Reimbursement for Physician Services:* Applying Current Procedural Terminology and HCPCS. Chicago: American Health Information Management Association.

LaTour, K. and S. Eichenwald Maki, eds. 2010. *Health Information Management: Concepts, Principles, and Practice,* 3rd ed. Chicago: American Health Information Management Association.

Odom-Wesley, B., D. Brown, and C. Meyers. 2009. *Documentation for Medical Records.* Chicago: American Health Information Management Association.

Sayles, N. and K. Trawick. 2010. *Introduction to Computer Systems for Health Information Technology.* Chicago: American Health Information Management Association.

Schraffenberger, L.A. 2012. *Basic ICD-9-CM Coding.* Chicago: American Health Information Management Association.

Shaw, P. and C. Elliott. 2012. *Quality and Performance Improvement in Healthcare,* 5th ed. Chicago: American Health Information Management Association.

Secondary References from Answer Key Rationales

Anthony, W.P., P.L. Perrewe, and K.M. Kaemar. 1996. *Strategic Human Resource Management.* Orlando: Harcourt Brace & Company.

Cohen, P.A. (1992) Meta-analysis: Application to clinical dentistry and dental education. *Journal of Dental Education* 56(3): 172–175.

Greenleaf, R.J. 1991. *Servant Leadership.* Mahwah, NJ: Paulist Press.

Hickman, C.R. 1990. *Mind of a Manager, Soul of a Leader.* New York: John Wiley and Sons.

Hogan, R. and R.B. Kaiser. 2004. What we know about leadership. *Review of General Psychology* 9(2):169–180.

Jennings, M.C. 2000. *Health Care Strategy for Uncertain Times.* San Francisco: Jossey-Bass.

Kempster, S. 2006. Leadership learning through lived experience: A process of apprenticeship? *Journal of Management and Organization* 12(1):4–22.

Kotter, J.P. 1995. Leading Change: Why transformation efforts fail. *Harvard Business Review* 73(2):59–67.

Kotter, J.P. 1990. *A Force for Change: How Leadership Differs from Management.* New York: Free Press.

Korabik, K. 1990. Androgyny and leadership style. *Journal of Business Ethics* 9:283–292.

Mathis, R.L. and J.H. Jackson. 2002. *Human Resource Management: Essential Perspectives.* 2nd ed. Cincinnati: South-Western Publishers.

McWay, D.C. 2003. *Legal Aspects of Health Information Management.* Clifton, NY: Delmar.

Medical Records Institute (MRI). 2002. *Healthcare Documentation: A Report on Information Capture and Report Generation.* Boston: Medical Records Institute.

Miller, R.D. 1986. *Problems in Hospital Law.* Rockville, MD: Aspen.

Norton, R., S. Kaplan, and P. David. 2000. Having trouble with your strategy? Then map it. *Harvard Business Review* 78 (Sept.–Oct.). http://hbr.org/2000/09/having-trouble-with-your-strategy-then-map-it/ar/6.

Peter, L.J. and R. Hull. 1969. *The Peter Principle: Why Things Always Go Wrong.* New York: William Morrow and Company.

Price-Waterhouse v. Ann B. Hopkins. 1987. Supreme Court of the United States. No. 87-1167. http://www.usdoj.gov/osg/briefs/1987/sg870104.txt.

Powers, V.J. 1997. Benchmarking study illustrates how best-in-class achieve alignment, communicate change. *Communication World* 14(2):30–33.

Pozgar, G.D. 2007. *Legal Aspects of Health Care Administration.* Sudbury, MA: Jones and Bartlett.

Rob, P. and C. Coronel. 2009. *Database Systems: Design, Implementation, and Management,* 8th ed. Boston: Course Technology, Thomson Learning.

Tichy, N.M. 1983. *Managing Strategic Change: Technical, Political and Cultural Dynamics.* New York: John Wiley & Sons.

Vroom, V. and P. Yetton. 1971. *Leadership and Decision Making.* Pittsburgh: University of Pittsburgh Press.

Zaleznik, A. 1977 (May–June). Managers and leaders: Are they different? *Harvard Business Review* 55:68–78.

Formulas

Hospital Statistical Formulas Used for the RHIA Exam

Average Daily Census

$$\frac{\text{Total service days for the unit for the period}}{\text{Total number of days in the period}}$$

Average Length of Stay

$$\frac{\text{Total length of stay (discharge days)}}{\text{Total discharges (includes deaths)}}$$

Percentage of Occupancy

$$\frac{\text{Total service days for a period}}{\text{Total bed count days in the period}} \times 100$$

Hospital Death Rate (Gross)

$$\frac{\text{Number of deaths of inpatients in period}}{\text{Number of discharges (including deaths)}} \times 100$$

Gross Autopsy Rate

$$\frac{\text{Total inpatient autopsies for a given period}}{\text{Total inpatient deaths for the period}} \times 100$$

Net Autopsy Rate

$$\frac{\text{Total inpatients for a given period}}{\text{Total inpatient deaths} - \text{unautopsied coroners' or medical examiners' cases}} \times 100$$

Hospital Autopsy Rate (Adjusted)

$$\frac{\text{Total hospital autopsies}}{\text{Number of deaths of hospital patients whose bodies are available for hospital autopsy}} \times 100$$

Fetal Death Rate

$$\frac{\text{Total number of intermediate and/or late fetal deaths for a period}}{\text{Total number of live births} + \text{intermediate and late fetal deaths for the period}} \times 100$$

Neonatal Mortality Rate (Death Rate)

$$\frac{\text{Total number of newborn deaths for a period}}{\text{Total number of newborn infant discharges (including deaths) for the period}} \times 100$$

Maternal Mortality Rate (Death Rate)

$$\frac{\text{Total number of direct maternal deaths for a period}}{\text{Total number of obstetrical discharges (including deaths) for the period}} \times 100$$

Caesarean-Section Rate

$$\frac{\text{Total number of caesarean sections performed in a period}}{\text{Total number of deliveries in the period (including caesarean sections)}} \times 100$$